Achieving Sterility in Medical and Pharmaceutical Products

DRUGS AND THE PHARMACEUTICAL SCIENCES

A Series of Textbooks and Monographs

edited by

James Swarbrick
Applied Analytical Industries, Inc.
Wilmington, North Carolina

ADDITIONAL VOLUMES IN PREPARATION

Achieving Sterility in Medical and Pharmaceutical Products

Nigel A. Halls

Glaxo Manufacturing Services
County Durham
United Kingdom

Marcel Dekker, Inc.　　　　New York•Basel•Hong Kong

Library of Congress Cataloging-in-Publication Data

Halls, Nigel A.
  Achieving sterility in medical and pharmaceutical products / Nigel
A. Halls.
      p. cm. — (Drugs and the pharmaceutical sciences ; 64)
  Includes bibliographical references and index.
  ISBN 0-8247-9014-6 (alk. paper)
  1. Sterilization. 2. Drugs—Sterilization. I. Title.
II. Series.
  [DNLM: 1. Sterilization—methods. 2. Drug Contamination-
-prevention & control. 3. Equipment and Supplies.   W1 DR893B v. 64
1994 / WA 240 H193a 1994]
RA761.H29 1994
614.4'8—dc20
DNLM/DLC
for Library of Congress   94-6372
                                                                    CIP

RA761
.H29
1994

The publisher offers discounts on this book when ordered in bulk quantities. For
more information, write to Special Sales/Professional Marketing at the address
below.

This book is printed on acid-free paper.

MARCEL DEKKER, INC.
270 Madison Avenue, New York, New York 10016

Current printing (last digit):
10 9 8 7 6 5 4 3 2 1

PRINTED IN THE UNITED STATES OF AMERICA

Preface

The purpose of this book is to help practitioners in the field who manufacture sterile products, pharmaceutical products, and medical devices to understand what needs to be done to achieve sterility. It is not intended for experts in specific sterilization technologies; indeed, that would necessitate a multivolume, multiauthor work.

Achieving sterility is an important aspect of quality assurance. In the pharmaceutical industry, quality assurance is most often dominated by personnel in analytical chemistry. In the medical device manufacturing industries, engineers tend to be most strongly represented. Real expertise in sterilization, particularly in sterilization science, is often concentrated among a limited number of microbiologically qualified staff who have gained their knowledge through hands-on experience of specific technologies. This book attempts to cover a wider spectrum of sterilization technologies than most practitioners might ever encounter in a working lifetime with one company or organization. It is intended to increase the breadth of knowledge of the sterilization specialist beyond the boundaries of his or her hands-on experience and to assist in communicating the fundamentals of the main sterilization technologies to interested personnel who work in this area but do not have a strong microbiological background.

A further purpose of this book is to bridge the knowledge gap for students and recently qualified graduates who may be moving or wishing to move into the sterile products manufacturing industries. There are few sources of information on achieving sterility lying between the general academic texts on microbiology and the level of detail and minutiae contained in advanced research papers, reviews, and guidelines on specific technologies.

Nigel A. Halls

Contents

Achieving Sterility in Medical and Pharmaceutical Products

1

The Need for Sterility

Why are some medical products required to be sterile? What distinguishes these products from other medical products that are not required to be sterile? What are the consequences of nonsterility?

Sterility is defined academically as the total absence of viable life forms. Some parts of the human body are always exposed to and contaminated by other forms of life. For instance, the external surfaces of the body, skin, hair, airways, etc., are unavoidably in contact with the general (microbiologically contaminated) environment. The buccal cavity and intestinal tract are regularly brought into contact with food- and water-borne microorganisms ingested with the diet. In many cases, some of these microorganisms colonize the surfaces of the human body and exist in harmony with the human host, sometimes even beneficially. Internal tissues are, however, expected to be totally free from microbial contamination.

The external surfaces of the "normal," fit, healthy human being have evolved to be effective barriers against penetration by opportunistic microorganisms to internal tissues that might provide them with nourishment at the expense of the host. Sometimes the external physical barriers fail, and then other antimicrobial defense mechanisms come into play, the immune system for instance. These internal mechanisms are combating infection. The various symptoms of infectious disease are the result of the interaction between the attempts by the infecting agent to colonize the internal tissues of the body and the attempts by the body's defense mechanisms to overcome this invasion.

From the sterility standpoint, no distinction can be made between the microorganisms that are known to be specific causative agents of disease and those that are not. It would of course be a major disaster if a specific pathogen such as *Bacillus anthracis* (the causative agent of anthrax) were to be introduced into the human (or animal) body through the administration of a supposedly therapeutic agent. On the other hand, microorganisms that are frequently found on man or in man's immediate environment are often assumed to be harmless because they are not associated with any specific disease. However, this is a wholly invalid assumption once the body's antimicrobial defensive barriers are broken down, as they usually are in the administration of parenteral preparations. These microorganisms may often be opportunistic pathogens. This is particularly applicable in the case of weak and debilitated patients who are ill-equipped to resist infection, even from microorganisms that have not evolved to be specially invasive. Complete freedom from all microorganisms is the only criterion for sterility.

Many therapeutic procedures quite deliberately break down the body's external physical barriers. From the application of an ointment or cream to broken skin, to simple or complex surgery, to injection, to implantation of, say, a cardiac pacemaker, all of these procedures risk infecting the patient by breaking through the body's external physical barriers. Infection will only occur, however, if these procedures carry viable microorganisms to internal tissues. On the other hand, if the devices and substances that are brought into contact with internal tissues are free from viable microorganisms—in other words, "sterile"— there ought to be no infection. This is the first and most fundamental reason why some medical products are required to be sterile.

There are other reasons.

Devices that are intermediates in the delivery of therapeutic substances to internal tissues, say infusion sets or catheters, ought to be sterile. It is quite obviously inappropriate to convey a sterile fluid from its sterile reservoir to internal tissues by a nonsterile route.

Garments, gloves, drapes and other operating theater paraphernalia ought to be sterile to prevent transfer of microorganisms to exposed internal tissue during surgical procedures.

Ophthalmic preparations, eye drops and eye ointments, ought to be sterile. There are three basic reasons for this. First, the cornea and other transparent parts of the eye have a particularly poor supply of blood and therefore a less responsive immune reaction than other parts of the body. Second, the transparency of these parts of the eye may be irreversibly damaged as a result of infection, with resultant permanent loss of vision. Third, infectious damage to the optic nerve is irreparable.

Numerous items of laboratory equipment, for instance pipettes, petri dishes, tissue culture plates, etc., have to be sterile. It is not within the scope of this text to address these, except to indicate striking similarities or differences in passing. In medical laboratory sciences particularly, containers for collection of tissues and body fluids for diagnostic analysis ought to be sterile. This is to ensure true results. Microbial contamination may pervert biochemical test results. Microbial contamination in containers may prevent accurate diagnosis of infectious conditions.

Numerous other medical products are not required to be sterile. Medicines to be taken by mouth, enemas, inhalations, most topical products, etc., need not be sterile. In some cases there may be a need to ensure that these products are microbiologically "clean," or free from specific pathogens or from microbiological contamination indicators, but there is no obligation to sterility.

Sterility is, however, required in some unusual circumstances for medical and nonmedical products that would not normally be associated with this type of need. For instance, you may consider sterile diets for hospital patients who are being treated with immunosuppressive therapeutic agents.

The scale of manufacture/preparation of sterile medical products and the complexity of sterile products is extremely wide ranging. Nothing is truly typical, nor can any text claim to be genuinely comprehensive. In this text we shall be addressing industrial manufacture of sterile products because governmental regulatory agencies and other ethical purchasing organizations have led industry to a certain consistency of approach that allows sensible generalizations to be made.

I. STERILE PHARMACEUTICAL PRODUCTS

Although it is conceivable that there are occasions when almost any pharmaceutical product may be required to be sterile, there are only two broad groups of sterile pharmaceutical products, parenteral products and ophthalmic products.

The *European Pharmacopoeia* is particularly succinct in its definition of preparations for parenteral use. It states that they are sterile preparations intended for administration by injection, infusion, or implantation into the human or animal body. Further, parenteral preparations are supplied, according to the *European Pharmacopoeia,* in glass ampoules, bottles, or vials, or in other containers such as plastic bottles or bags or as prefilled syringes.

This colorless but clear definition of parenteral products has pretty well universal acceptance and is likely almost timeless as well: current United States FDA thinking is that no new forms of presentation of sterile parenteral products are likely to be approved without strong justification of their being of benefit to the patient. Commercial reasons are not acceptable.

Nonetheless, there is a huge variety and wide range of parenteral products. Some parenteral dosage forms may be filled into their presentation forms or systems of containment under controlled but nonsterile conditions and then exposed to a sterilization process; these are referred to as terminally sterilized products. Terminal sterilization must be the method of first choice for all sterile pharmaceutical products. This is good sense and reflects current FDA thinking. There are a variety of terminal sterilization processes, thermal, chemical, or by ionizing radiation, but quite frequently dosage forms cannot withstand any of these treatments without loss of efficacy. In these cases, recourse is made to aseptic manufacture. With aseptic manufacture, product contact components making up the system of containment are sterilized before filling; the dosage form is sterilized before filling, preferably by filtration but possibly by some chemical treatment that may or may not be part of its initial synthesis, and the whole final presentation is filled and sealed in a sterile or as near sterile as possible environment.

The first broad division among parenteral products is between those used for infusions and those used for other forms of administration. Infusions are principally intended for administration in large volumes and are frequently referred to as large volume parenterals (LVPs). With the exception of sterile *Water for Injection,* LVPs are usually made to be isotonic with blood, for example saline, dextrose, etc.

The widest range of parenteral products are however, the small volume parenterals (SVPs). These may be sterile solutions for injecting directly into the patient. They may be concentrated solutions or suspensions or emulsions or even solids (solid dosage forms may be anhydrous, crystalline, or freeze dried [lyophilized]) for dilution or reconstitution in LVPs for direct injection or infusion into the patient.

Table 1 lists some examples of sterile parenteral products classified as LVPs or SVPs, as aseptically filled or terminally sterilized, and as solutions, suspensions, or solid dosage forms.

The therapeutic application of sterile parenteral products is almost boundless. Some products can only be administered via the parenteral route; others may be administered orally, as suppositories, intranasally, etc. This begs the

Table 1   Some Examples of Sterile Parenteral Products

Product	Condition	Achievement of Sterility
LVPs		
Water for Injection USP	"Solution"	Terminal (steam)
Dextrose Injection USP	Solution	Terminal (steam)
SVPs		
Ranitidine Injection USP	Solution	Aseptic fill
Suxamethonium Chloride Injection BP	Solution	Terminal (steam)
Progesterone Injection BP	Solution	Terminal (dry heat)
Epinephrine Oil Suspension USP	Suspension	Aseptic fill
Sterile Ceftazidime USP	Solid	Aseptic fill
Diamorphine Injection BP	Solid (lyophilized)	Aseptic fill

question of why they are being manufactured for parenteral administration at all. The answer may lie with the product's efficacy, with the acuteness of the condition it is being used to treat, or with the speed at which relief of symptoms is required.

Taking the products listed in Table 1, Ceftazidime has only two entries in the USP, *Ceftazidime for Injection* USP and *Sterile Ceftazidime* USP. Both are restricted to parenteral administration because of loss of efficacy when delivered by other routes.

Ranitidine, on the other hand, has entries as *Ranitidine Injection* USP and *as Ranitidine Tablets* USP. Epinephrine has entries as an inhalation aerosol, an injection, an inhalation solution, a nasal solution, an ophthalmic solution, and an oil suspension.

The question of which Ranitidine preparation to use for ulcer treatment is based primarily on the acuteness of the condition and with regard to convenience for maintenance therapy after the condition has been brought under control. Parenteral administration is in the main restricted to acute symptoms under hospital supervision; oral administration is used for maintenance of the condition once stabilized.

Epinephrine is rather more complicated, because it may be used in connection with a variety of symptoms. Subcutaneous or intramuscular injection may be life-saving for anaphylactic shock or acute allergic reactions, or it may

be used to control bronchial spasm in acute attacks of asthma. The other preparations are used for local application in less extreme circumstances. For
instance, the ophthalmic solution may be used for pupillary dilation in connection with ophthalmic treatment or glaucoma.

Sterile Epinephrine Ophthalmic Solution USP takes us out of the realm of
sterile parenteral products into ophthalmics. The manner of presentation of
ophthalmics (i.e., as drops or ointments) is likely to be quite familiar. For the
most part (but not exclusively) they are in multidose presentations. As such,
most formulations include some form of preservative to control proliferation of
any microorganisms that may by chance contaminate the product on one or other
of the occasions when it is open, or during the time when it is left standing on the
bathroom shelf. The inclusion of preservatives in a multidose formulation of an
ophthalmic (or parenteral) is not a primary part of the process of achieving
sterility. It has quite a separate purpose.

Even when preservatives are included in single-dose presentations (as they
often are), their efficacy against particular types of microorganisms can never be
legitimately used as an excuse for tolerating in-process contamination by preser-
vative-sensitive types. Nor can the inclusion of preservatives in products be
used to shorten or reduce the intensity of sterilization processes applied to products or their containers to lower than normal levels of sterility assurance. Preservatives are supplementary, not intrinsic to industrial-scale processes of achieving
sterility.

An important distinction to draw between sterile parenteral products and
sterile ophthalmic products concerns pyrogens. We will discuss pyrogens in
some detail at a later stage in this text. They are substances that induce fever
when injected into mammals. As such, all sterile products for parenteral administration are expected to be pyrogen free, and if dilution is required they must be
diluted in a sterile pyrogen-free diluent. The tie-up between sterility, absence of
pyrogens, and administration by injection is reflected in the USP distinction
between the two types of water recommended for ingredient purposes, *Purified
Water* and *Water for Injection*. The former is not required to be pyrogen free,
and only the latter is to be recommended for use in preparations intended for
parenteral administration.

Sterile ophthalmic products have no requirement to be pyrogen free.

II. STERILE MEDICAL DEVICES

The term *medical device* includes instruments, apparatus, implements, con-
trivances, implants, or other similar or related articles used in medical treatment.
A medical device does not achieve its principal intended purpose through chemical or pharmacological action within or on the body. Some medical devices need
to be sterile.

For the most part (measured as numbers of devices used per annum), sterile medical devices are for single use only ("use once and then discard"). Hypodermic products and infusion sets are probably the most familiar types of single-use medical device. They are a comparatively modern concept that had its origins in economics and in an increasing concern over hospital-acquired infections in the "antibiotic era." Before the 1950s, most medical devices were washed, resterilized, and reused repeatedly. As antibiotics became widely available in that decade, "background" infections diminished in proportion to those that were associated with the reuse of equipment. At the same time the cost of labor for reprocessing was increasing while the cost of plastics was decreasing. Single-use industrially sterilized plastic medical devices grew from a practical alternative to be the current norm.

There are a huge range of different types of medical device. Approval to market is, as with pharmaceuticals, subject to regulatory control. Most sterile devices in the U.S.A. would require premarket approval and fall into Class III of Part 860 of the *Code of Federal Regulations.* This classification places great emphasis on devices that are life-supporting or life-sustaining, or those that are of substantial importance in preventing impairment of human health, or those that present potential unreasonable risks of illness or injury.

Less formally, sterile devices may be classified in terms of the severity of the consequences of their nonsterility.

(a) Devices making no direct contact with patients. Mainly we are thinking here of diagnostic devices, bearing in mind that contamination could affect the patient through adversely influencing the outcome of the diagnostic process.

(b) Devices that contact intact external surfaces, such as sterile dressings, or heavily contaminated internal surfaces such as the gut, for instance examination gloves. Patients are not really likely to die as a result of nonsterility of these products unless a chance contaminant has unusually invasive properties competitive with the innate microflora. Their sterility is of greater significance with susceptible patients, an example being those with severe burns, where infection is a major and possibly life-threatening issue. The range of products in this category is impossible to exemplify, but it may be of value to consider sterile cellulosic dressings. Almost inevitably, cellulosics are microbiologically contaminated, often with bacterial endospores, and therefore pose a severe challenge to whatever sterilization process is being applied.

(c) Devices that contact directly or indirectly with the intravascular system, say "giving" sets. Here we are talking about a vastly important route of administration, often for severely ill patients. The consequences of microorganisms being delivered directly to the blood, with the risk of them being carried throughout the body and inducing generalized infection, is self-evident. The principal portion of a "giving" set is tubing, possibly rubber but nowadays more likely extruded plastic tubing. The temperatures reached in plastic extrusion processes are quite high enough to bring about significant reductions in numbers of vegetative microorganisms. However, cooling in water and subsequent assembly and packing may lead to recontamination.

(d) Invasive devices. This category probably contains the largest number of items marketed, because it embraces hypodermic needles and syringes, scalpel blades, catheters, etc. These are the mechanisms that break down the body barriers. If we take hypodermic syringes as an example of this type of device, we can consider a variety of different types of manufacturing technology versus their effects on microorganisms. The characteristic single-use disposable hypodermic syringe is made up of three pieces; the barrel, the plunger, and the plunger tip ("stopper"). Plastic plungers and barrels are almost always injection-molded; rubber "stoppers" are compression-molded. The temperatures achieved with these technologies kill most microorganisms. Like "giving" sets, contamination may occur during assembly and packaging; the numbers and types of microbial contaminants on packaged hypodermic syringes prior to sterilization are very largely related to the number of manual steps involved in these processes. In modern automated high-volume manufacture the final biological challenge *(bioburden)* on these products tends to be quite low [1].

(e) Implantable devices. Some of these may have a purely mechanical function, like the very widely used artificial hip- and knee-joints; others have more complex and life-sustaining functions, such as cardiac pacemakers. In both cases there is a critical necessity for sterility. Again the technologies of manufacture and the complexity of the devices are diverse. The technology of manufacture of cardiac pacemakers is that of the electronics industry, where cleanliness is of the highest importance to function as well as to the control of bioburden. The technology of manufacture of artificial hip-joints is the technology of the machine shop, casting, milling etc. Cleanliness is an additional constraint to the traditional practice of these crafts.

As with sterile pharmaceuticals, pyrogens are of significant importance to medical devices. Any device intended for administration of a sterile parenteral pharmaceutical must (like the pharmaceutical preparation) be pyrogen free. So must all invasive and implantable devices.

III. CONSEQUENCES OF NONSTERILITY

Hospital-acquired (nosocomial) infections are not uncommon. However, those that have been conclusively attributed to supposedly sterile but actually nonsterile pharmaceutical products or medical devices are quite rare. The consequences of these incidents have not confined themselves to the companies responsible for the failure to achieve sterility but have reverberated throughout the whole "steriles" industry. No company wishes to face the litigation, loss of sales, loss of goodwill, and generally bad publicity that accompanies nonsterility. Most of all, ethical companies are in the business of preserving life, not in the business of killing people—and death is often the consequence of nonsterility.

Although all the incidents described below occurred quite a long time ago and technology has changed and improved, and regulatory control has become more demanding and explicit, we believe that because sterility can only be achieved consistently by constant vigilance there are important lessons to be learned from reviewing them again.

A. The 1971/72 Devonport Incident in the U.K.

The Devonport Incident occurred in the U.K. Some postoperative patients who had been given supposedly sterile but actually contaminated infusion fluids died; others made unnecessarily long recoveries. The incident summarized below is described fully in a U.K. government enquiry, the *Clothier Report* [2].

A series of untoward reactions were seen among postoperative patients in the Devonport Section of Plymouth General Hospital in March 1972. Seven patients were involved; five died. A commonality among the patients was that all had received intravenous administration of *Dextrose Injection* BP (5% dextrose infusion fluid). All intravenous infusion fluids containing dextrose were promptly withdrawn from use, and samples were examined in the laboratory.

A batch of bottles of "sterile" *Dextrose Injection* BP manufactured by Evans Medical Ltd. (at that time a major U.K. producer of these types of products) was found to be contaminated by *Klebsiella aerogenes* and other gram-negative coliform bacteria. Approximately one-third of all of the bottles from the incriminated batch were found to be nonsterile. The concentration of bacteria in the bottles of fluid was sufficiently high to be visually perceptible to the naked eye; this would typically mean more than 10^6 bacteria per mL.

An urgent investigation was initiated. The possibility of other batches being contaminated could not be ruled out, and all Evans Medical infusion fluids were placed under U.K. government embargo.

The contaminated product was traced to incorrect operation of Evans Medical's sterilizing autoclaves. The Committee of Enquiry [2] concluded that too many people believed that sterilization of fluids was easily achievable with simple equipment operated by men of little skill under a minimum of supervision.

What had happened was this. The sterilization process for bottles of *Dextrose Injection* BP was by exposure to saturated steam at a temperature of 116°C (specified as 240°F) for 30 min. Evans Medical's autoclaves were equipped with two temperature measuring devices. The first and most important of these was a recording thermometer located in the chamber drain. This is normally the coolest part of any autoclave, and it is from the sensor located at this point that the decision should be made that the autoclave has reached its specified operating temperature and exposure timing begun. The second temperature measuring device on the autoclaves was a dial thermometer located near the steam inlet pipe at the top of the chamber. This location usually reaches high temperatures more rapidly than any other location in the chamber. The recording thermometers in the chamber drains of Evans Medical's autoclaves were subject to faulty operation, and it had become "custom and practice" for the sterilizer operators to give more credence to the dial thermometers. It had been quite common for batches of autoclaved infusion fluids to be released as sterile despite the temperature recorder chart showing an inadequate cycle.

The batch implicated in the Devonport Incident had been sterilized in April 1971. The recording thermometer did not indicate the expected rise in temperature. On past experience, the manager of the area ignored this device and continued the process through reliance on the dial thermometer. With hindsight it is possible to conclude that all of the air had not been vented from the bottom of the chamber at the beginning of the cycle and consequently the correct operating temperature was not being achieved throughout the load; particularly it was not being achieved for bottles in the lower part of the chamber nor in the chamber drain. In other words, the recording thermometer had been operating correctly. If the correct procedure had been followed the process would not have been approved nor allowed to continue.

It is not pertinent to go into the detail of the likely technical problems that may have led to stratification of steam over air in the bottom of this autoclave, but details are given in the *Clothier Report* [2].

The contaminated bottles were not detected by end-product sterility testing. The batch was released to a wholesaler and distributed to the Devonport Section of Plymouth General Hospital in March 1972. The high concentrations of microorganisms found in the infusion fluid can be attributed to the period of time between sterilization, distribution, and final administration to the patients.

B. The 1970/71 Rocky Mount Incident in the U.S.A.

The Rocky Mount Incident, which began in July 1970, affected at least 378 patients in at least 25 US hospitals [3,4]. Forty patients died.

As with the Devonport Incident, the Rocky Mount Incident was caused by contaminated bottles of infusion fluids. The fluids were all made by Abbott Laboratories in their Rocky Mount, North Carolina, plant. The company's infusion products were recalled in March 1971.

The clinical features seen with patients who received these contaminated fluids included extreme fever, shaking chills, systemic toxicity, abdominal cramps, nausea, vomiting, diarrhea, delirium, and seizures. With hindsight these are the symptoms of gram-negative septicemia, but with sudden onset they were sometimes misdiagnosed [3]. Confirmed cases were mainly drawn from large hospitals, often university teaching hospitals, using significantly large volumes of infusion fluids. It is possible that many more patients in small hospitals were implicated, but the cases were not diagnosed or reported.

The microorganisms associated with the epidemic were identified with *Enterobacter cloacae*, *Enterobacter agglomerans*, and other *Enterobacter* species. The precise cause of the incident was traced to a program of gradual replacement of Gilsonite cap liners for the infusion fluid bottles with an elastomer cap liner (Fig. 1). The replacement program was operating only in Abbott's Rocky Mount plant and not on any other Abbott operating site.

Felts et al. [4] examined 93 bottles containing a variety of different infusion fluids. They looked for microbiological contamination of the closures.

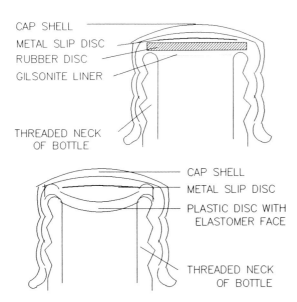

Fig. 1 Simplified drawings of bottle cap differences in Rocky Mount Incident (not to scale).

Twenty-five bottles were contaminated; all were made at Abbott's Rocky Mount plant, and all had elastomer cap liners.

None of the twenty bottles from Abbott's North Chicago plant were contaminated; all had Gilsonite cap liners. Neither of two bottles from batches made at the Rocky Mount plant with Gilsonite cap liners was contaminated.

The study also showed that dye could penetrate from closures with elastomer cap liners into infusion fluids in the course of normal usage. No dye penetration was seen in bottles with Gilsonite cap liners. It was also shown in experimental conditions that the types of microorganisms implicated in the epidemic and found on contaminated closures could increase to concentrations of up to 10^6 per mL in Abbott's 5% Dextrose, Normal Saline, and Water for Injection products.

What seems to have happened was that the elastomer-lined caps became contaminated after sterilization. Investigations showed that tap water used in cooling could readily penetrate the interstices of the screw thread and get into the cap assemblies. These microorganisms most likely got into the fluids when the bottles were being set up for infusion, through removal and replacement of the cap, through shaking the bottle to distribute additives throughout the fluid, or through seepage during the time the bottles were hanging inverted for infusion.

The principle that the Rocky Mount Incident exemplifies is the criticality to achieving sterility of even the seemingly most trivial change in components or methods or what have you. The concept is validation—demonstrating that a changed process is capable of doing what it is supposed to be doing. In this case the change of cap liner had not been demonstrated to be capable of maintaining sterility, and lives were lost.

C. The 1972/73 Cutter Laboratories Incident in the U.S.A.

In March 1973, Cutter Laboratories withdrew from the market all 1,000-mL bottles of 5% Dextrose in Lactated Ringers Injection produced at its Chattanooga, Tennessee, plant since September 1972. Five cases of clinical septicemia had been associated with administration of these fluids; three of the five patients died [5].

The microorganisms implicated in the clinical cases were *Enterobacter agglomerans*, *Enterobacter cloacae*, and *Citrobacter freundii*. Unopened bottles from the same plant were found to be contaminated with the same and similar microorganisms, in some instances to the point of visible turbidity.

This incident is cited here only as an indication that there have been other incidents similar to the two main examples described above. Nonsterile parenteral products have a real potential to kill. Death is a quite probable consequence of administration of nonsterile parenteral products, so that achieving sterility for these products concerns the sanctity of human life.

D. The 1964 Imported Eye Ointment Incident in Sweden

Postoperative infections after ophthalmic surgery may arise from any one of several sources. In 1964, eight patients in two Swedish hospitals developed *Pseudomonas aeruginosa* infections from contaminated hydrocortisone eye ointment [6].

The consequences were total blindness in the infected eye of one patient, considerable loss of vision in two patients, and reduced visual acuity in the remaining five patients.

The levels of *Pseudomonas* contamination in unopened tubes of ointment from the batch that had been implicated in the infection, and in other batches from the same manufacturer, were higher than 2,000 colony-forming units per gram. The isolate was resistant to neomycin and amphomycin, the two antibiotics included in the formulation.

The ointment had not been terminally sterilized. It had been manufactured aseptically, no preservatives were included in the formulation, and the manufacturers had laboratory data to show that microbial growth in the ointment was very unlikely due to the low water content and the presence of two antibiotics in high concentrations.

In the case of this ointment, the petrolatum base was dry heat sterilized in bulk prior to the addition of solubilized active ingredients. Evidently a film of water had condensed on the surface of the cooling petrolatum and this had become contaminated by *Pseudomonas aeruginosa* shown to be present on towels, shoes, gloves, and hands of personnel engaged in manufacture of the ointment. The contaminant was shown by simulation to be capable of multiplying in the film of moisture over periods of storage similar to those that might have arisen routinely in practice.

Antibiotic-resistance may have developed over time in the premises.

E. The 1981 Imported Indian Dressings Incident in the U.K.

This incident of contaminated first aid dressings was detected by regulatory vigilance [7]. No patient infection arose. The U.K. regulatory authorities were alerted to the possibility of supposedly sterile first aid dressings of Indian manufacture being contaminated from reported concern in Australia.

Thirty-three of 38 batches of Indian dressings were found to be contaminated by aerobic spore-forming bacilli; levels of contamination by these microorganisms were typically less than 10 per dressing. Low levels of contamination by *Clostridium* sp and by fungi were also seen. The spore formers and clostridia were attributed to inadequate steam sterilization [8]. Because the fungal contamination was heaviest in the outer part of the dressings, and because there was visual evidence of the paper wrappings having been wet at one time, it was assumed that this had arisen from poststerilization contamination.

The U.K. official report on this incident [7] concluded that the contaminating microorganisms were of low pathogenicity. They also commented that the types of first aid dressings involved were most commonly applied to wounds that were already contaminated. They evaluated the risk to health arising from use of these contaminated dressings to be small. Nonetheless they severely criticized the manufacturers for labelling these products as "sterile" and judged the risk to be unacceptable.

F. Incidents Originating from Other Sources

It should not be assumed that all serious consequences arising from the use of nonsterile products are of industrial origin. Many are from products prepared and sterilized in hospital pharmacies. Those which have been confirmed to be of industrial origin are usually more widespread because of the scale of manufacture and distribution. A few examples are included below to indicate the range of problems encountered over many years.

Michaels and Ruebner [9] reported two cases of patients whose temperatures rose dramatically while receiving intravenous therapy and then settled normally when the infusion apparatus was taken down. These authors attributed these reactions to in-use contamination of giving sets left in place over several days and over several changes of bottles of infusion fluid.

In 1969, cracks in bottles led to inadvertent infusion of fungal-contaminated glucose-saline solution to two patients [10]. Fungal microcolonies were visible in the fluids. Both patients recovered satisfactorily after prompt treatment with ampicillin and amphotericin B.

In the latter half of 1971, 40 patients in a U.K. hospital acquired bacteremia, urinary tract infections, or respiratory infections from in-house manufactured sterile parenteral solutions. The infective agent, *Pseudomonas thomasii,* was traced to water used for cooling sterilized parenteral solutions in a rapid-cooling autoclave. The microorganism had penetrated beneath the cap seals and entered the bottles of fluid either in the autoclave or when the caps were disturbed on setup [11].

Postoperative eye infections from contaminated instruments, fluids, and eyedroppers have been periodically reported over many years [12,13,14]. *Pseudomonas aeruginosa* and *Serratia marcescens*, among other microorganisms, have been implicated. Some permanent visual impairment was common.

REFERENCES

1. Halls, N. A., Joyce, T. M., Doolan, P. T., and Tallentire, A. (1983). The occurrence of atypically high presterilization microbial counts ("spikes") on hypodermic products. *Radiation Physics and Chemistry* **22** (3–5): 663–666.

2. *Report of the Committee Appointed to Inquire into the Circumstances, Including the Production, Which Led to the Use of Contaminated Infusion Fluids in the Devonport Section of Plymouth General Hospital* (C. M. Clothier, Chairman). London: Her Majesty's Stationery Office, 1972.

3. Felts, S. K., Schaffner, W., Melly, A., and Koenig, M. G. (1972). Sepsis caused by contaminated intravenous fluids—Epidemiological, clinical and laboratory investigation of an outbreak in one hospital. *Annals of Internal Medicine* **77** (6): 881–890.

4. Maki, D. G., Rhame, F. S., Mackel, D. C., and Bennet, J. V. (1976). Nationwide epidemic of septicemia caused by contaminated intravenous products. *American Journal of Medicine* **60**: 471–485.

5. Center for Disease Control (1973). Follow-up on septicemias associated with contaminated intravenous fluids. *Morbidity and Mortality Weekly Report* **22** (13): 115–116.

6. Kallings, L. O., Ringertz, O., Silverstolpe, L., and Ernerfeldt, F. (1966). Microbial contamination of medical preparations. *Acta Pharm. Suecica* **3**: 219–228.

7. Marples, R. R. (1983). Contaminated first-aid dressings: Report of a working party of the PHLS. *Journal of Hygiene* (Cambridge) **90**: 241–252.

8. Thomas, S., Dawes, C. E., and Hay, N. P. (1981). Microbiological contamination of imported wound dressings. *Pharmaceutical Journal* **1981**: 783.

9. Michaels, L. and Ruebner, B. (1953). Growth of bacteria in intravenous infusion fluids. *Lancet* **1953**: 772–774.

10. Robertson, M. H. (1970). Fungi in fluids—A hazard of intravenous therapy. *Journal of Medical Microbiology* **3**: 99–102.

11. Phillips, I., Eykyn, S., and Laker, M. (1972). Outbreak of hospital infection caused by contaminated autoclaved fluids. *Lancet* **1972**: 1258–1260.

12. Lepard, C. W. (1941). *B. pyocyaneus* ulcer. Report of three cases: Results of sulfapyridine therapy in one case. *Transactions of the American Academy of Ophthalmology and Otolaryngology* **46**: 55–60.

13. Ayliffe, G. A. J., Barry, D. R., Lowbury, E. J. L., Roper-Hall, M. J., and Martin Walker, W. (1966). Postoperative infection with *Pseudomonas aeruginosa* in an eye hospital. *Lancet* **1966**: 1113–1117.

14. Templeton, W. C., Eiferman, R. A., Snyder, J. W., Melo. J. C. and Raff, M. J. (1982). *Serratia* keratitis transmitted by contaminated eyedroppers. *American Journal of Ophthalmology* **93**: 723–726.

2
Sterility and Sterility Assurance

Sterility is defined as the total absence of viable life-forms (Table 1). The concept of sterility is absolute and acknowledges no boundaries. However, life-forms are ubiquitous on this earth, and sterile conditions can only exist within some form of boundary. Once these boundaries are broken down the sterile condition is inevitably lost.

Sterile conditions exist in nature—within solid rock for instance. But should the rock be broken open it will become nonsterile unless this is done within some other set of barriers that protect the rock's internal sterility. Sterile conditions will exist in the heart of a volcano, protected by temperatures

Table 1   Definition of Terms Used in Chapter 2: Sterility and Sterility Assurance

Term	Definition
Sterility	Condition in which an item is totally free of all life-forms
Viable (of microorganisms)	Capable of reproducing to discernable levels
Discernable level (of viable microorganisms)	*Either* as a colony, film, or slime visible to the naked eye or under the microscope on solid nutrient media, *or* as a physical or chemical change (usually turbidity) in the composition of fluid nutrient media
SAL (Sterility Assurance Level)	The probability of a supposedly sterile item being contaminated by one or more micro-organisms
Validate (of a sterilization process)	Demonstrate that the process is capable of achieving what it is supposed to achieve

destructive to the essential molecules of life. In this case the barriers protecting sterility are barriers of heat; nonsterile conditions will exist outside these barriers.

In real terms, sterility is therefore a descriptive and limited concept. A sterile item is one that does not contain, carry, or harbor any viable life-forms. The sterile item must be protected from contamination from the general environment; otherwise it becomes nonsterile.

Thus far the concept of sterility is still academic in that we have not addressed the question of how sterility or (conversely) nonsterility can be identified or demonstrated for an item. The situation then becomes immediately murkier. No method exists whereby an item can be examined and be shown conclusively to be sterile. All methods approach the problem from the viewpoint of demonstrating nonsterility; if nonsterility cannot be demonstrated, the item is therefore assumed to be sterile. This is not necessarily true.

I. DETECTION OF NONSTERILITY

Demonstration of nonsterility has its origins in the very beginnings of microbiology as a science in the eighteenth and nineteenth centuries. In those times there was considerable debate over the origins of microorganisms ("animalcules")—by spontaneous formation (spontaneous generation) from non-living materials, on the one hand, versus formation from living "seeds" or "germs," which were supposed to be always present in the atmosphere, on the other.

Pasteur produced some pretty conclusive evidence in favor of the germ theory through his famous swan-necked flask experiments. This experimentation was based upon detection of microorganisms by visible changes in organic infusions. The infusions were boiled up in the flasks, and as long as measures were in place to prevent microorganisms from entering the flasks from the atmosphere, the infusions remained clear to the naked eye, and microbial growth was undetectable on microscopic examination. If the necks were broken off, the infusions became turbid to the naked eye, and microorganisms became detectable under the microscope. Pasteur was using growth or absence of growth in organic infusions as a method of distinguishing between the sterile and the nonsterile states.

Considering Pasteur's turbid organic infusions in more detail, we can enlarge upon the concept of viability, which features as a qualification within the definition of sterility. Viability has various meanings for different life-forms; in this text we are concerned with viability among microorganisms, a concept quite different from viability when used in connection with mammals, for instance. For a microorganism to be viable, it must have the capability of reproducing itself, in practice not just once but through sufficient successive divisions to form a colony on solidified nutrient media or visible growth in fluid nutrient media. In these terms, Pasteur's turbid organic infusions were quite clearly nonsterile.

But can we reasonably infer that Pasteur's clear organic infusions were necessarily sterile? The answer to this question is not straightforward. The clear infusions were clearly not contaminated by any microorganisms that had the capability of reproducing in these media under the conditions within which they were incubated. The question remains whether there might have been microorganisms present that if transferred to another medium, or incubated under different conditions, would have multiplied to discernable levels. Naturally this question is now unanswerable.

The general point to be made is that detectable microbial growth in any test system is positive confirmation of nonsterility, but absence of growth can only give an assurance of sterility limited by the conditions of the test. It is fundamental that sterility for an item can never be confirmed with 100% certainty by any test method.

A. Compendial Methods of Detecting Nonsterility

In essence, the pharmacopoeias are compendia of end-product specifications for therapeutic substances and descriptions of methods approved for testing substances against these specifications. Methods for detecting nonsterility were introduced into the *British Pharmacopoeia* in 1932 and into the *United States Pharmacopoeia* in 1936. In the years since, the methods have changed in detail and in application, and have differed between the two major pharmacopoeias.

Table 2   Evolution of the Test for Sterility in the British Pharmacopoeia

1932	Media and methods specified, direct inoculation, incubation at 37°C for 5 days
1948	Thioglycollate medium included as an alternative recovery medium for anaerobes
1953	No change from 1948
1958	Accommodation made for solid dosage forms, "neutralizers" allowed, and specified for certain antibiotics
1963	Incubation conditions changed to 30–32°C for 7 days, membrane filtration allowed for certain antibiotics
1968	Sample sizes included to allow certification of batches as sterile
1973	Inclusion of European Pharmacopoeia 1971, recommended that the membrane filtration technique be used wherever possible, inclusion of media control tests; incubation conditions changed to 30–35°C for bacteria and 20–25°C for fungi over 7 days
1980	General expansion of the detail
1988	No significant change from 1980

Therefore, although the concept of sterility is absolute and unchanging, the standard required to confirm its achievement has never been consistent.

Consider the development of the *Test for Sterility* in the *British Pharmacopoeia* since 1932 (Table 2). The test in 1932 was an appendix of only two paragraphs. It described the media to be used in the test and a method of testing.

From this first compendial method it was recognized that the selection of appropriate media was imperative to the detection of as wide a range of microorganisms as possible. Replicate samples were required to be tested in each of two fluid media. The first of these, intended for recovery of aerobic microorganisms, was defined as meat extract containing 1% peptone, and the pH after sterilization was required to be in the range 7.2 to 7.8. Recovery of anaerobic microorganisms was recommended in the same medium but with the addition of heat-coagulated muscle to a depth of 1 cm at the bottom of the tube.

The recommended method was to inoculate the preparation directly into each of the two media, taking care that the final concentration of any phenolic antiseptic in the preparation under test was diluted to less than 0.01%. Media were to be incubated at 37°C for 5 days.

The 1932 BP method recommended that the complete contents of a container should be tested only when the volume was less than 2 mL (two equal parts, one part for each medium). For volumes of 2 mL and greater, 1 mL was to be tested in each medium.

If there was no growth under these conditions, the preparation was confirmed as sterile (passed the *Test for Sterility*). If growth was detected, retests and second retests were allowed on fresh samples. The preparation could only be failed if growth was seen in all three tests, or if the same microorganisms were found in two of the tests.

The presentation of the *Test for Sterility* in **BP** 1932 was in the same style as any of the other chemical or physical test methods in the pharmacopoeia, i.e., without any guidance on the number of items from a batch of items required to make up a valid sample.

Three themes contained in the BP 1932 *Test for Sterility* merit some emphasis.

(a) The test presumed sterility. Even with the limitations of the sterilization technology of the 1930s, the pharmacopoeia was presuming sterility unless nonsterility could be convincingly and conclusively demonstrated. This is rather unusual because it goes against the grain of scientific criticality to assume that a hypothesis is valid unless it can be proven otherwise. The test was far less a critical test for sterility, as one might suppose it was intended to be, than a test for nonsterility—i.e., false nonsterile results were thought to be more likely than false sterile results (the pharmacopoeia had more faith in the potential of the recommended media to recover microorganisms than it had in the ability of laboratories to perform successful aseptic manipulations).

(b) The test did not address total freedom from microorganisms for preparations in 2 mL volumes or greater. For these larger volumes it was really a microbial limit test with a lower sensitivity of detection of one microorganism per mL.

(c) The test gave no guidance on interpretation of data from replicate recovery conditions.

These three themes, which are common to the BP, USP, and other pharmacopoeias, remain fundamentally unchanged up to and including the current editions of the compendia, despite numerous other modifications and alterations to broaden recovery conditions and improve methods.

After 1932 very little changed in the next edition, BP 1948, except for the introduction of an alternative medium for recovery of anaerobes, a medium very similar in composition to present-day *Thioglycollate Medium* USP. The BP *Test for Sterility* remained at about two paragraphs in this edition and in its 1953 edition.

By 1958 the test increased in complexity by accommodating solid dosage forms and antibiotics. The weight separating those solid dosage presentations for which the total contents were to be tested and those for which only a portion was to be tested was 100 mg. For preparations of 100 mg or more, only 50 mg was to be tested in each medium. Less than 100 mg, equal parts were to be divided between the two media. Substances to "neutralize" microbial growth inhibitors were allowed to be included in test media. Details of neutralizers were given for various antibiotics.

In BP 1963 there were two important innovations: incubation changed from 37°C for 5 days to 30–32°C for 7 days, and a membrane filtration technique was introduced for certain antibiotics.

The membrane filtration technique, now almost universally used for pharmaceutical preparations but not for devices, was an advance of major significance. BP 1963 advised dissolution of the antibiotic in saline, followed by passage through a sterile membrane filter. The principle is that soluble substances pass through the membrane in solution and any microbial contaminants are retained. The membrane was to be cut in two and one half tested for aerobic microorganisms and the other for anaerobes. This technique is more amenable to all of the contents of a single presentation being tested, and also, if necessary, for the contents of several presentations to be bulked and tested together in one set of media.

Only in 1968 does the BP provide any guidance on the number of items (2% of the total containers or 20 containers, whichever is the fewer) that should comprise a sample whereby the result of the *Test for Sterility* can be extended to apply to batches of product needing to be certified as sterile. These sampling requirements only reflected those given in the UK *Therapeutic Substances Regulations* [1] that had existed since 1952. Importantly it was a move away from the straightforward specification of a test method that had predated it.

The *Tests for Sterility* in the 1973, 1980, and 1988 revisions of the *British Pharmacopoeia* are greatly expanded from earlier editions, with up to five pages to include control systems ensuring that test media are themselves sterile and capable of supporting microbial growth, and that substances under test do not inhibit the growth of selected microorganisms. The conditions became 30–35°C for bacteria and 20–25°C for fungi over 7 days incubation since 1973 onwards.

Through all these changes the three flawed themes described above remain unchanged: as a means of confirming sterility the test is flawed because it presupposes sterility rather than nonsterility; in many cases it operates only as a microbial limit test; and it avoids addressing the interpretation of data obtained from replicate samples in different media. Nonetheless, the two techniques of the compendial sterility tests (direct inoculation and membrane filtration), the consideration given over many decades to broad-spectrum microbial recovery conditions, and the recommendations concerning media control together provide a very powerful basis for a method of detecting nonsterility if that is what is required.

B. Newer Technologies

The speed of response from compendial methods of testing for nonsterility is limited by the incubation period. Of course, it often happens that a nonsterile item will produce discernable growth within 24 or 48 h under compendial conditions: to demonstrate the converse, i.e., that an item is sterile, the test must run through its allotted incubation period.

The food industry has invested a considerable amount of effort and expertise into the development of quicker methods of detecting microorganisms. So far none of these have found application to sterility/nonsterility as it is understood in the pharmaceutical and medical products industries. This is because the main drive from the food industry has been toward microbial limit tests based on the presupposition that some microorganisms will always be present in most products. Where microorganisms are required to be totally absent, e.g., *Clostridium botulinum* from canned foods, the food industry has recognized the inadequacy of end-product testing and relies on verification of a rigorous process specification. The presupposition of the pharmaceutical and medical products industries is that viable microorganisms are in fact absent from sterile products and the purpose of the test for nonsterility is only to confirm this. This presupposition is much harder to reconcile, both philosophically and technically.

Data from newer technologies is challenging even the basic assumptions of the traditional definition of viability and the compendial approach to determining nonsterility. Many types of common microorganisms, including *E. coli, Salmonella,* and *Streptococcus faecalis* [2,3] have been shown to be capable of developing viable but nonculturable forms in stressed environments.

The first source of evidence for the existence of viable but nonculturable microorganisms is from the newer technologies of detection. Typically this is where counts of microorganisms by newer technologies fail to correlate with counts by culture methods, or exceed counts obtained by culture methods. The issues of viability and culturability are of course always challengable on the basis of there being always another set of culture conditions not studied and of the application of the newer technology being overzealous.

However, the definition of viable but nonculturable microorganisms has been in the main based on pathogens that have been shown to be capable of growth in warm-blooded hosts while defying recovery by microbiological culture techniques. There is a particularly striking epidemiological example of this [4] in which treatment against *Campylobacter* of the water supply to a chicken shed resulted in the disappearance of a particular serotype from the chicken population even though it had not at any time been recovered by culture techniques from the water supply.

Summaries of the main applications of newer technologies to detection and enumeration of microoganisms merit consideration.

1. Determination of Microbial ATP: ATP is present in all living cells. The concentration of ATP decreases through phosphorylation reactions that occur when microorganisms lose their viability. Methods for detecting microorganisms based on ATP determination presume that the presence of detectable levels of ATP confirms the presence of viable microrganisms, and conversely the absence of ATP confirms the absence of viable microorganisms.

ATP can be detected through a luminescent reaction catalyzed by an ATP-specific enzyme:

$$E + ATP + LH_2 \rightarrow E\text{-}LH\text{-}AMP + PP$$
$$E\text{-}LH\text{-}AMP + O_2 \rightarrow E\text{-}L\text{-}AMP + H_2O_2 + light$$

where LH_2 is luciferin, an oxidizable substance obtained from fireflies that after reaction with ATP becomes the substrate for an oxidative reaction catalyzed by an enzyme, luciferase (E). The reaction results in production of light.

The intensity of light produced may be detected by a photomultiplier and related to the concentration of ATP present.

The amount of ATP in vegetative bacterial cells can be expected [5] to be around 10^{-13} to 10^{-12} mg, less in spores, more in yeasts. The lower limit of the sensitivity of the technique is usually quoted to be on the order of 10^{-10} mg. This value may be even higher if background ATP has to be taken into account. The technique has two difficulties, therefore, for the detection of nonsterility—low sensitivity and the possibility of false alarms (false positives) due to extraneous ATP.

2. Detection of Changes in Electrical Resistance: Viable microorganisms metabolize. End-products of metabolism, when released into the surrounding media, cause detectable changes in electrical resistance. Detection of these changes is the basis of several well-developed conductance, impedance, and capacitance methods of detecting microorganisms.

In the main, these types of instruments have been used to determine numbers of microorganisms in nonsterile milieux. A sample of the preparation under examination would typically be incubated in an appropriate growth medium contained within an electrode-equipped well. Changes in electrical resistance (conductance, impedance, and/or capacitance) can be monitored and recorded during incubation, or alternatively instruments can be set to a threshold value linked to a lower sensitivity of detection. With commercially available instruments the threshold of detection has usually been quoted at around 10^7 microorganisms per mL. For enumeration of microorganisms, the incubation time required to reach the threshold "trigger" is inversely proportional to the initial concentration of microorganisms in the sample.

The absolute lower limit of sensitivity of methods based on electrical resistance and existing technologies is somewhere around 10^2 microorganisms per sample versus background effects. This is really too insensitive for detection of nonsterility. Furthermore, there are significant media-to-media, batch-to-batch, and microorganism-to-microorganism differences in sensitivity. Media recipes that have stood the test of time for growth promotion may contain electrically active substances that make them totally unsuitable for detection of microorganisms via resistance changes. Some microorganisms may even in the best of circumstances give only minimal changes that are not detectable against the background. Optimal conditions for one microorganism may not be optimal for another. So overall these methods lack the robustness of traditional approaches for detecting broad-spectrum nonsterility, and they leave some doubt about the absence of a response confirming sterility.

3. Near-Infrared Spectrometry: Near-infrared spectrometry is an exciting new technology for detecting microorganisms in fluids. The principle is based on scattering of near infrared light by solid objects in fluids; suspended microorganisms by absorption at wavelengths between 1100 and 1360 nm; microorganisms adhering to container walls by absorption in the region of 1600 to 2200 nm.

Research with deliberately contaminated intravenous infusion bags [6] has demonstrated lower limits of detection of around 10^2 colony-forming units per mL of fluid. Some distinction between different types of microorganisms was also indicated. Whereas these recently published limits of sensitivity would be wholly unsatisfactory to the detection of nonsterility (and conversely the confirmation of sterility), the near infrared approach has the advantage over other existing methods of being noninvasive and nondestructive. With development, this technology could add an extra dimension to existing microbial-detection practices.

II. CONFIRMING STERILITY OF BATCHES BY END-PRODUCT TESTING

Sterility is an attribute. An item can exist in only one of two conditions, sterile or nonsterile. Methods are available (see above) for testing items to determine in which of these states the item exists. All technologies involve sacrificing the item or at the very least compromising its sterility. After testing, the item is no longer in a sterile useable state. Therefore the value of testing an item must lie with the item being a sample or part of a sample from a greater population or universe about which we are trying to gain information.

This was the principle that led to the pharmacopoeias adding sampling schemes to the basic method of the *Test for Sterility*. As mentioned previously, the original pharmacopoeial entries comprised a simple test method applicable to finding out whether items tested were nonsterile. Sampling schemes appeared in the U.K. *Therapeutic Substances Regulations* in 1952, in the USP in 1955, and in the BP in 1968. The actual sample size has varied, usually related to a percentage of the number of containers in the batch but limited to a maximum sample size (Fig. 1).

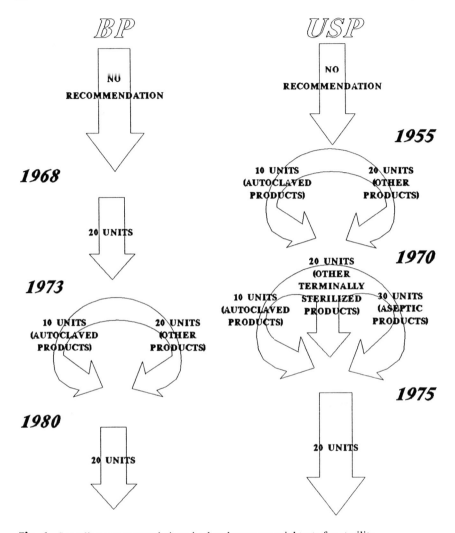

Fig. 1 Sampling recommendations in the pharmacopoeial tests for sterility.

With the introduction of sampling schemes, the compendial *Tests for Sterility* became approved methods for confirming the sterility of batches of supposedly sterile products by means of end-product testing.

As a means of confirming sterility, all pharmacopoeial sampling schemes for the *Test for Sterility* are totally inadequate. This has been well known at least since the 1940s [7].

The usual sample size is 20 items. Imagine a batch of 100 items of which only 99 were sterile. This would be totally unacceptable for release if the single nonsterile item were known to be present. But the odds are in favor of that batch passing a pharmacopoeial sterility test. Divide the batch into five sets of twenty and consider how many of those samples would pass the *Test for Sterility*. Four would pass and only one would fail. If the sample tested contained the contaminated item, then the retest sample would not contain a contaminated item—so the batch would be passed as sterile.

The formal statistics surrounding this are not complicated [8,9,10]. The probability of drawing n consecutive sterile items from a population of items is given by the expression

$$(1 - p)^n \tag{2.1}$$

where p = the proportion of nonsterile items in the population and n = the number of items in the sample.

Conversely, the probability of selecting one or more nonsterile items in a sample of n items is given by the expression

$$1 - (1 - p)^n \tag{2.2}$$

Annex 1 describes the use of these expressions to calculate the effectiveness of the pharmacopoeial *Test for Sterility* as a means of confirming sterility. Quite simply, the test does not confirm sterility. Batches of product released on the basis of a *Test for Sterility* alone could too easily contain significant proportions of nonsterile items.

The inadequacies of the *Test for Sterility* are acknowledged in the pharmacopoeias themselves. The *European Pharmacopoeia* does not have a long history of publication; three of its four fascicules carry a "disclaimer" to the *Test for Sterility*. Only in 1971 did the EP publish an unembellished method description and sampling plan. Each of its next revisions, EP 1978, EP 1980, and EP 1986 start their sections headed *Test for Sterility* with an italicized paragraph stating the following:

(a) . . . a satisfactory result (from the *Test for Sterility)* only indicates that no contaminating microorganism has been found in the sample examined in the conditions of the test.

(b) . . . extension . . . to the whole of a batch . . . requires the assurance that every unit in the batch has been prepared in such a manner that it would also have passed the test. Clearly this depends on the precautions taken during manufacture.

(c) . . . (for) products sterilised in their final sealed containers physical proofs, biologically based and automatically documented, showing correct treatment throughout the batch during sterilisation are of greater assurance than the sterility test.

(d) (The *Test for Sterility*) . . . is the only analytical method available to the various authorities who have to examine a product for sterility.

The same messages appear, but initially less explicitly stated, in all revisions of the USP since USP XVIII (1970) under the heading of *Sterilization.* USP XX (1980), Section <1211> introduces the very direct statement, "The sterility test is intended as the official referee test in the event that a dispute arises concerning the sterility status of the lot."

In summary, end-product testing is not a defendable option, either scientifically or officially, for confirming the sterility of batches of supposedly sterile products.

III. CONFIRMING STERILITY BY COMPLIANCE WITH PROCESS SPECIFICATIONS

If sterility cannot be confirmed by end-product testing, one alternative is that it may be confirmed by some positive affirmation that every item in a batch of product has been treated by some officially recognized process. An appropriate analogy might be the hard-boiled egg. Imagine that any method of testing boiled eggs for hardness must be destructive. So rather than boiling eggs for arbitrary lengths of time and periodically sampling we could decide to boil for 20 min, and so the definition of a hard-boiled egg by its process specification is any egg that has been held in boiling water at 100°C for 20 min.

Table 3 lists the sterilization cycle specifications currently recognized by the three major pharmacopoeias ("compendial cycles"). A body of knowledge exists to support the view that products that are properly exposed to any one of these compendial cycles will be free from all viable microorganisms. The origins of the compendial cycles are lost in history except to say that they were probably based on available technology (121°C is achieved by saturated steam held at a pressure of 15 lbs per inch^2, which is equivalent to 1 bar or one atmosphere).

There are two points to be considered in relation to compendial cycles. The first is common to all approaches to sterility control: there must be reliable assurance of every treated item in the batch having been exposed to the specified parameters that deliver lethality. The second point is that compendial cycles do not take account of any differences in the numbers and types of microorganisms contaminating the product before treatment. Returning to the analogy of a hard-boiled egg, definition by process specification would embrace everything from a quail's egg to an ostrich's egg being hard-boiled by holding in water at 100°C for 20 min.

Table 3 Current Compendial Sterilization Cycles

Sterilization process	Cycle specification	Reference	Comments
Saturated steam	15 min at 121°C	EP (1983), BP (1988), and USP XXII (1990)	For aqueous preparations
			When "auto-claved" is stated in the monograph
	3 min at 134°C	BP (1988)	For dressings
Dry heat	30 min at 180°C | 1 h at 170°C | 2 h at 160°C |	EP (1983) and BP (1988)	
Gamma radiation	2.5 Mrads (25 kGy)	BP (1988) and USP XXII (1990)	
Filtration	Passage through a 0.22 μm membrane	EP (1983), BP (1988), and USP XXII (1990)	

There have been huge technological advances in contamination control during manufacture and in precise control of sterilization processes since most of the compendial cycles first came to be recognized. Under these changing circumstances it has not made sense to many sterilization scientists and practitioners to standardize a definition of sterility on something as rigid as a process specification. This has led to the concept of sterility assurance that now appears alongside the *Test for Sterility* and the compendial cycles in all the major pharmacopoeias.

IV. STERILITY ASSURANCE

The concept of sterility assurance invokes the idea of confidence. How confident should we be that an item is sterile? All three of the major pharmacopoeias now require assurance of less than 1 chance in 1,000,000 that viable microorganisms are present in a sterilized article or dosage form (10^{-6} probability of nonsterility). To obtain this assurance we must have good knowledge of the effects of sterilization processes on microbial populations.

Microbial inactivation has been well researched. This is particularly true for populations of bacteria. Although each type of microorganism responds differently to the various available sterilization processes, the form of inactivation of microbial populations is broadly similar enough to depict a general case based on exponential death.

A. Exponential Inactivation

The death of a single microbial cell is a biochemical process (or series of processes); the entrapment of individual microbial cells in or on filters is due to physical forces. These effects on individual cells are peculiar to individual sterilization processes. On the other hand, the effects of inactivating processes and filtering processes on populations of microbial cells are sufficiently similar to be described by one general form—exponential death. Exponential kinetics are typical of first-order chemical reactions. For inactivation this can be attributed to cell death arising from some reaction that causes irreparable damage to a molecule or molecules essential for continuing viability.

For filtration it can be assumed that binding of the microorganism to the filter is due to interactive effects between molecules on the surface of the filter and molecules on the surface of the microorganisms, again first-order kinetics.

Chemical kinetics cannot be assumed for aseptic manufacture; nonetheless, protection of items from microbiological contamination in clean rooms can never be perfect and may therefore be assumed to be subject to the laws of chance. The sterility assurance concept is certainly applicable to aseptic manufacture, but not in a manner directly comparable to terminal sterilization processes.

For simplicity, the kinetics of exponential inactivation of populations of microorganisms will be illustrated by reference to the application of some form of inimical treatment to a pure culture of bacteria. There are plenty of data in the scientific literature to support the general case.

Let us suppose that the inimical process can be applied to a population of bacteria in an incremental manner. Initially and after various periods of exposure we can withdraw samples from the population and count the number of viable bacteria present. When we plot these data as a survival curve on arithmetic axes we get the form of Fig. 2a. The relationship of survivors to time of exposure shows an initial rapid decline and then levels out and becomes asymptotic to the time axis. If we were to convert the survivor data to logarithms and then plot these logarithmic data against time of exposure we would obtain a straight-line relationship (Fig. 2b). This is the general form for exponential or logarithmic survival curves.

There are two important related conclusions to be drawn from this general form of exponential or logarithmic inactivation

(a) The logarithmic axis has no zero point. Successive points on the axis become proportionately smaller, but zero can never be reached. What this means to sterilization processes is that you can never define a time of

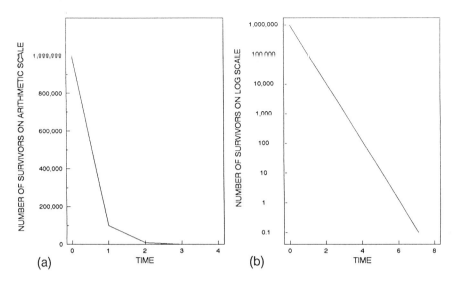

Fig. 2 Kinetics of microbial inactivation (generalized). (a) Arithmetic/arithmetic; (b) logarithmic/arithmetic.

exposure that will guarantee sterility in the sense of total absence of viable microorganisms.

(b) For each fixed increment of exposure time, a constant proportion of the surviving population is inactivated. If a particular exposure time decreases the number of viable microorganisms in a population by 90%, and that period of exposure is then applied to the survivors, it will again decrease the population by a further 90%, i.e., the number of survivors will be decreased to 10% by the first treatment, 1% by the second treatment, etc. The time of exposure required from a sterilization process to reduce a microbial population by 90% is called the decimal reduction value (*D*-value). *D*-values are specific for particular microorganisms but may differ for the same microorganism according to its condition during treatment.

But what does this mean to sterilization? Fig. 2b shows an initial population of 10^6 bacteria. After six equal increments of time (applied *D*-values) there is only one survivor (Fig. 2b). After seven *D*-values, the graph suggests that there is only one tenth of a bacterium left surviving, and common sense would suggest that single tenths of bacteria have no survival capability. In fact, what the graph tells us is that after application of seven *D*-values there is only a one-in-ten chance of a single intact bacterium surviving, after eight *D*-values a one-in-one-hundred chance of a single intact bacterium surviving, and so on.

In summary, there is always a finite probability of a survivor occurring, no matter the strength or duration of a sterilization process. In other words, absolute sterility, in the sense of total freedom from all viable life forms, can never be achieved in practice. The acceptance of exponential inactivation kinetics has led to two different approaches to the establishment of standards of satisfactory sterilization treatment, the inactivation factor approach and the sterility assurance level (SAL) approach.

1. Inactivation Factors ("Overkill"): When the canning industry addressed the question of how much heat treatment was needed to protect the public from botulism through ingestion of viable spores of *Clostridium botulinum,* they decided that twelve *D*-values was a safe level. In other words, they reckoned on a treatment that would reduce a population of spores of *Cl. botulinum* by a factor of one thousand billion.

The USP allows a very similar approach (termed "overkill") to the determination of valid sterilization processes for compendial preparations ("a lethality input of 12*D* may be used in a typical "overkill approach").

To adopt an overkill approach it is necessary to fix on a reference microorganism. In food canning, this was easily chosen—the toxin of *Cl. botulinum* is the single major hazard from canned products, and the spore of *Cl. botulinum* is considerably heat-resistant. For medical sterilization the situation is less clear; any microorganism could lead to a fatality. Microorganisms (biological indicators) used for this purpose are usually chosen to be among the most resistant types known against the chosen sterilization treatment. Spores of *Bacillus stearothermophilus* are generally recommended for sterilization by saturated steam. Other microorganisms are more appropriate for other sterilization processes.

There are both practical and academic problems associated with setting standards for sterility on the basis of inactivation factors.

In the first instance, the intensity or duration of the sterilization treatment may be very high, possibly too high to be tolerated by some products. This begs the practical question of why such an intense process must be used. It might be argued that the actual contaminants on the product are far less resistant to the sterilization treatment than the reference microorganisms.

Secondly, as with defining sterility in relation to process specifications, there is something incongruous about using the same treatment, in this case 12 *D*-values versus some reference microorganism, to all products regardless of the initial number and responsiveness of the actual contaminants.

2. Sterility Assurance Levels: The concept of the sterility assurance level (SAL) not only considers the kinetics of inactivation of microbial populations but also addresses the numbers of contaminants on product items prior to sterilization treatment. In some applications it may also take account of the resistance of actual contaminants to particular sterilization treatments and any effects that the condition of the product and its immediate environment may have on resistance.

An SAL is a target to be achieved for the treated product items. It is a probability. It is defined as the probability of a treated item remaining contaminated by one or more viable microorganisms.

The major pharmacopoeias, and most regulatory documents governing sterile medical devices, require an SAL of 10^{-6} or better (less than one chance in one million of an item being nonsterile after treatment) to be achieved for terminally sterilized products. Why 10^{-6} rather than 10^{-5} or 10^{-7}? This is not known.

The Canadian Standard for Industrial Sterilization of Medical Devices by the Steam Process, 1979 [11] differentiates between products intended to come into contact with compromized tissue, which are required to have an SAL of 10^{-6} (quoted as a probability of being sterile of 99.9999%) and products not intended to come into contact with compromized tissue, which are required only to have an SAL of 10^{-3} (a probability of being sterile of 99.9%). No other formally acknowledged exceptions to the general rule of sterility being defined as a 10^{-6} SAL are known.

SALs are not directly measureable. A supposedly sterile item can only be sterile or nonsterile, as indicated by testing or usage. Estimates of probabilities of nonsterility can be obtained by testing samples of item populations or universes of items that have been treated identically. For instance, if each item in a population has a probability of nonsterility of 10^{-1}, we will find that approximately one item in ten will be nonsterile, etc. The sampling dimensions required to support SALs of 10^{-6} by end-product testing are impossibly large for both routine and nonroutine purposes.

SALs for terminally sterilized products are substantiated (validated) by extrapolation of measurable responses of microbial populations at sub-process treatment levels to process treatments that ought to be providing the specified nonmeasureable SALs. Extrapolation can only be justified when a response takes a regular form and can be supported by theory. This is clearly the case for the kinetics of inactivation of microbial populations.

Simulation trials (media fills) do not validate SALs for aseptically filled products. The frequently encountered regulatory requirement for aseptic filling processes to be validated by simulation versus a standard of no more than 1 contaminated item in 1,000 items is not intended to imply that an SAL of 10^{-3} is satisfactory for these products. The SAL is a complex function of contamination rate and probability of survival; the simulation trial measures only the first of these factors. SALs for aseptically filled products are in all likelihood much better than 10^{-3}, only they are nonmeasureable, and there is no basis or generally accepted theory to support extrapolation.

The concept of the SAL specifies a single target for all sterilization processes. This takes account of the different initial levels of contamination that may be encountered for different products manufactured in different places and under different circumstances. This is its strength. Versus the other standards for sterility, it places far greater demands on sound knowledge of the product's bioburden (numbers and types of microorganisms contaminating the product prior to sterilization), its response to the sterilization treatment, and the uniformity of the particular sterilization processes. Ultimately it relies on the confidence in the extrapolation required to demonstrate that the process is capable of achieving what it is supposed to achieve.

V. DETERMINANTS OF STERILITY ASSURANCE

When validation depends on extrapolation, it is of utmost importance to have confidence in the base data from which the extrapolation is to be made. The determinants of sterility assurance are defined by an equation describing exponential inactivation. When time is the variable, as in Fig. 2b, the expression is written as

$$N_t = N_0 \cdot e^{-kt} \tag{2.3}$$

where N_t = the number of microorganisms surviving after time t, N_0 = the number of microorganisms prior to treatment, t = the time of treatment, and k = a constant expressing the resistance of the microorganisms to the particular sterilization treatment, i.e., a measure of the slope of the survival curve.

To determine an appropriate time t of treatment to achieve an SAL of 10^{-6} = N_t it is necessary to have a fix on the bioburden N_0 on the items prior to sterilization and the slope k of the dose/response curve. The term k is most usually expressed via the D-value, when the expression becomes

$$t = \frac{\log_{10} N_0 + \log_{10} SAL}{D} \tag{2.4}$$

The determinants of sterility assurance that must be considered in determining appropriate treatment levels to achieve particular SALs (in this text it will be assumed that the target SAL is 10^{-6}) or in validating existing treatment levels are, therefore, bioburden (microorganisms contaminating the item prior to treatment) and the shape and slope of the survival curve.

A. Bioburden

Bioburden is a jargon word that can assume at least two different meanings. As a determinant of sterility (N_0) it means each and every viable life-form contaminating the product item. As a practical concept it usually means an estimate of the numbers of microorganisms contaminating a product item, subject to all the usual limitations of microbiological technique. Any bioburden claimed to be a good estimate of N_0 is required to have been obtained from a fully validated procedure.

All practical bioburdens are estimates. Estimates of what? Usually they are measures of average, expressed as the mean number of colony-forming units per product item or per unit volume or per unit weight of the preparation. A good estimate of mean numbers of microorganisms per item will describe a typical item drawn randomly from the population. However, with every population of nonsterile items, there will be some degree of variation in numbers of contaminants from one item to another. Some items will possess fewer contaminants than would be deduced from the mean; others will possess more items.

Is it therefore proper to use the mean number of microorganisms contaminating an item prior to sterilization as a valid measure of bioburden in the sense of N_0? Alternatively, should the highest recorded number of colony-forming units per item be used as the estimate of N_0, or should the estimate of N_0 be the mean plus one or two or three standard deviations?

This issue was addressed by Doolan and coworkers [12] in 1985. Although their model was derived from experience with radiation sterilization, it is a general case for all forms of exponential inactivation. These authors considered the case of a sterilization treatment being applied to a population of items contaminated with a pure culture of microorganisms where the mean number of organisms per item was initially greater than one. At some level of treatment the mean number of survivors would drop to one per item, so that the total number of contaminating microorganisms would be equal to the number of items. At this level of treatment, the most unfavorable way, from a sterilization standpoint, in which the survivors could be distributed over items would be if each individual item were to have one contaminant. In such circumstances every item in the population would be nonsterile. If this number of microorganisms were to be distributed over the population of items in any other manner it would only lead to noncontaminated (sterile) items appearing in the population. They termed this most unfavorable distribution "the limiting case."

In the limiting case there are two phases associated with application of a sterilization treatment to a population of items with an initial mean number of contaminants greater than one. In the first phase the effect of increasing treatment is to decrease the total number of microorganisms without effecting any change in the proportion (P_{LC}) of nonsterile items in the population:

$$P_{LC} = 1$$

In the second phase, the mean number of contaminants begins to drop below one, and the proportion of nonsterile items also begins to drop below one. The effect of increasing dose beyond this point is to decrease this proportion such that always for the limiting case

$$\log_{10} P_{LC} = \log_{10} m \quad when \ m < 1 \tag{2.5}$$

where m = mean number of survivors per item. For microorganisms that respond to sterilization treatments according to the simple function $N_t = N_0 \cdot e^{-kt}$ (Eq. 2.3), the behavior of P_{LC} with increasing treatment is therefore completely independent of the initial distribution of microorganisms on items and is determined solely by m_0, the average number of microorganisms per item prior to treatment (Fig. 3).

The limiting case treatment for an SAL of 10^{-6} can be calculated from

$$t_{P_{LC}} = D(\log_{10} m_0 - \log_{10} P_{LC}) \tag{2.6}$$

or when $\log_{10} P_{LC} = -6$ for an SAL of 10^{-6}

$$t_{P_{LC}} = D(\log_{10} m_0 + 6)$$

where D = the D-value, the time required to reduce the number of survivors in a population by 90%, and $m_0 = N_0$, the average number of microorganisms contaminating the product prior to treatment.

These equations illustrate the importance of the mean number of microorganisms contaminating products prior to sterilization and show that SALs calcu-

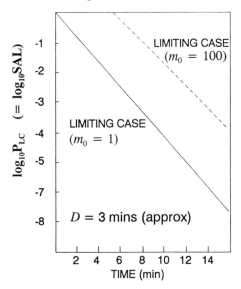

Limiting Case lines for two values of m_0 according to increasing time of treatment

Fig. 3 Limiting case model.

lated using the mean are not influenced by the occurrence of occasional high numbers of microorganisms contaminating the odd item in the population.

Finally, on theoretical considerations relating to bioburden, most experimental work on sterilization kinetics has addressed the inactivation of pure cultures of microorganisms. Most "real life" bioburdens are mixed cultures. An important assumption surrounding the application of experimental pure culture situations to practical mixed culture situations is that each component of a mixed culture should behave independently of the others. As far as is known there is no evidence to doubt this assumption.

1. Determination of Bioburden: Estimates of bioburden are no better than the microbiological techniques used for their determination. There is no single standard approach for dosage forms for medical devices. Therefore all techniques tend to be particular, and generalizations are difficult to make.

With medical devices, the first stage in bioburden determination is to remove microorganisms from the device and suspend them in a fluid diluent for subsequent manipulation.

Removal of microorganisms from devices usually requires some means of counteracting the forces that retain them on the device [13]. In the simplest technologies, devices may be flushed through with diluent. They may be shaken, either manually or mechanically after immersion in diluent. They may be sonicated. These techniques should not be inimical, and it may be convenient to complete a composite validation technique for physical removal and for the effects of the diluent.

Removal of microorganisms from the product is less complicated for liquid and soluble pharmaceutical dosage forms. Removal and recovery methods are those of the microbial limit tests contained in the compendia. Liquid dosage forms are passed through 0.45 μm membrane filters and flushed with a diluent or a diluent plus neutralizer if the dosage form is antimicrobial. The membranes are plated on suitable media and incubated to recover viable contaminants. Weighed amounts of soluble solid dosage forms are dissolved at about 1:10 in a diluent, filtered, flushed, and plated. When products are heavily contaminated, microbial recovery may be by direct plating methods rather than membrane filtration. Many laboratories still prefer to use membrane filtration techniques in these cases even if secondary dilution is required.

The first issue in bioburden determination that merits validation is the choice of fluid used in preparatory stages of removal of microorganisms from devices and for suspending, dissolving, and diluting dosage forms. Phosphate buffer pH 7.2, buffered sodium chloride–peptone solution pH 7.0, and lactose broth are recommended in the various compendia. Saline, Ringer's solution, and 0.1% peptone water are also quite commonly used. These fluids should neither promote the growth of microorganisms nor inhibit their growth. The compendia suggest *Staphylococcus aureus, Pseudomonas aeruginosa, E. coli, Salmonella,*

Bacillus subtilis, and Candida albicans for validating microbial limit tests and by inference for validating diluents, etc. The addition of local isolates should be considered.

The second stage in bioburden determination is the recovery of microorganisms in culture. For both medical devices and pharmaceuticals (as stated above), the methods of choice are membrane counts and plate counts. Soybean casein digest agar is recommended for pharmaceutical dosage forms. In a survey of bioburden recovery methods used with medical devices [14], most laboratories appear to use either variations on soybean casein digest agar or variations the American Public Health Association's standard methods media recommended for plate counts of microorganisms in milk and dairy products. Incubation times range from 2 to 21 days; temperatures are usually in the range 30 to 37°C.

Recovery conditions should also be validated against a range of microorganisms as described above. Variation in recovery characteristics of laboratory media should be guarded against through application of rigorous batch-to-batch quality control techniques.

B. Survival Curves

Beside bioburden, the other determinant of sterility assurance is the survival curve and its shape and its slope. It is not correct to assume that all survival curves are of the simple linear type when data is plotted on semilogarithmic graph paper. Three general types of survival curve have been reported, the exponential curve, the "shouldered" curve, and the "tailed" curve (Fig. 4).

1. Technical Considerations: Survival curves cannot be derived theoretically for particular microorganisms versus particular sterilization treatments; they can only be determined through laboratory studies.

If it is assumed that the technology of the sterilization treatment in question can be controlled sufficiently well to deliver reasonably precise incremental treatment levels, then the procedures and precautions required to derive reproducible survival curves are quite similar.

Most survival curves have been constructed for pure cultures of microorganisms. Reproducible curves, however, will not be obtained unless cultures are genetically homogeneous, physiologically homogeneous, and free from clumps. Assurance of genetic homogeneity resides with sound microbiological technique. Physiological homogeneity demands that all cells within the population are at the same stage in their growth cycles and have been grown in the same media under the same conditions of incubation. Microorganisms respond quite differently to sterilization treatments according to their physiological state; in the grossest case the bacterial endospore responds quite markedly differently to sterilization treatments than the vegetative cell of the same microorganism. Microorgan-

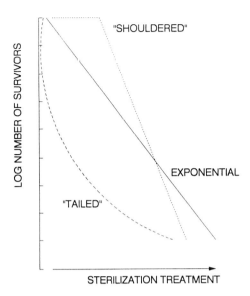

Fig. 4 The range of general types of survival curves.

isms bound together within films or slimes may be protected from penetration of the lethal effects of particular sterilization treatments. More importantly, clumping may affect the number of survivors counted after treatment. Most survival curves have been constructed for microorganisms exposed in aqueous suspension (including saline, inorganic buffers, etc.) or dried onto a surface (e.g., membrane filters, glass cover slips, capillaries).

Equal in importance to the condition of the microorganisms is the means of estimating the numbers of microorganisms surviving incremental sub-process sterilization treatments. The characteristic approach to counting microorganisms over the whole general field of microbiology is the plate count. Many survival curves have been wholly or partly derived from plate count data. However, the technique in the form of direct plating is only useful for concentrations of microorganisms greater than about 20 per mL. Membrane filtration may increase the sensitivity of colony counting by about a factor of ten. Confident extrapolation of survival curves to SALs of 10^{-6} or thereabouts would normally require data covering lower probabilities of survival than can be achieved with colony counts. Data of this type is usually obtained from quantal response experiments.

In quantal response experiments data is only recorded as good or bad, plus or minus, pass or fail. In the case of sterility, quantal response experiments set out to detect nonsterility, normally by sterility test techniques. Replicate samples are individually tested and, after incubation, scored as sterile or nonsterile. For a set of replicates, the proportion nonsterile (proportion positive) is a measure of the probability of occurence of a nonsterile item (the SAL). This approach is not economical with samples if low probabilities of nonsterility are being targeted. It is also subject to a lower limit of sensitivity set by practical considerations. The frequency of spurious results in aseptic transfers attributed to accidental laboratory contamination (false positives) is usually quoted [15] as being around 10^{-3} (Borick and Borick [16] reported supportive data: 30 of approximately 60,000 sterility tests on materials known to be sterile were found to be contaminated in testing).

Figure 5 summarizes the limits of sensitivity of the methods used in the construction of survival curves. Plate count methods only yield meaningful results when the number of microorganisms per sample tested is greater than about ten; quantal response methods do not come into play until the probability of occurence of nonsterility falls below 1 (below 100%) and are limited by false positives to SALs greater than 10^{-3}.

To make valid extrapolations from exponential survival curves it is useful not only to obtain as much sensitivity as possible but also to cover as wide a range as possible. This should be at least through three, preferably four, log

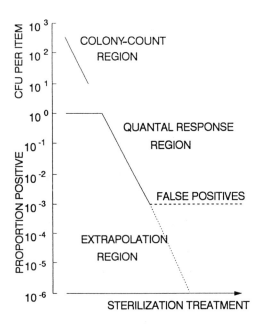

Fig. 5 Construction of a survival curve from various methods of obtaining data, subject to their limitations.

cycles. With laboratory studies of pure cultures of microorganisms this should only rarely be a problem. However, since the 1980s there has been some considerable interest in constructing survival curves for the innate contaminant microflora on actual product items (often as mixed cultures). With some very clean products, for instance hypodermic needles for which the average number of contaminants per item prior to sterilization is usually less than 1, it may not be easy to cover a reasonable range of inactivation versus a lower limit of sensitivity of an SAL of 10^{-3}. To some extent this may be resolved by multiitem quantal response experiments, i.e., incubation of several items together in one culture.

Estimates of the probability of occurrence of nonsterile items can be obtained from such data through an expression derived from the binomial distribution [17]. Suppose a population of items is contaminated with from 0 to n microorganisms per item. A proportion of microorganisms will harbor one or more microorganisms; therefore any random item taken from the population can be designated to have a probability q of being free from microorganisms (sterile) and a probability p of carrying one or more microorganisms.

Assuming that the nonsterile items are randomly distributed throughout the population, then the probabilities of there being 0, 1, 2, etc., nonsterile items in a random sample of n items drawn from the population are given by successive terms of the binomial expansion:

$$(q + p)^n = q^n + (n)q^{n-1}p + (n)q^{n-2}p^2 \cdots \qquad (2.7)$$

Thus q^n represents the probability of such a sample containing no contaminated items. Conversely, $1 - q^n$ is the probability that a sample of n items contains one or more contaminated items.

For any series of quantal response data, the ratio of nonsterile items (growth) to sterile items (no-growth) after incubation is an estimate of the term $1 - q^n$. This estimate in turn allows calculation of q and p. Importantly, p is a measure of the probability of an item being nonsterile.

An example of how this calculation may be used is given in Annex 2.

A final laboratory issue connected with mixed cultures is how to handle multiple media data [17]. The compendial methods of testing for sterility have long advocated the use of replicate media and incubation conditions to ensure recovery of as wide a range of microorganisms as possible. It is recognized that any one recovery condition is not absolutely selective for a particular kind of microorganism, and it is to be expected that on occasions the same kind of organism will be recovered in more than one condition. On the other hand, there will be occasions when a single particular recovery condition will only be suitable for the recovery of a particular kind of organism: if this condition were not part of the test it could be falsely presumed that no viable microorganisms were present.

When it comes to determining survival curves there is no need to consider multiple media unless the curve addresses naturally mixed cultures within which each component has not been or cannot be precisely identified. However, any studies with naturally contaminated products ought to use multiple media.

Doolan and coworkers [18] used three compendial recovery conditions to construct survival curves for naturally contaminated medical devices: soybean casein digest medium incubated at 20–25°C, the same incubated at 30–35°C, and fluid thioglycollate medium incubated at 30–35°C for 14 days. Three tests for sterility therefore constituted the basis for observing the presence of viable microorganisms in three replicate conditions making up one sample.

Their problem was how to interpret the data. Table 4 illustrates some results from this type of experiment. The data are scored as "net positives": media are coded as replicates before incubation, and then, after incubation, one net positive is scored for any one, two, or three growths in the replicates making up a single sample. In Table 4, the proportion positive obtained from net positives is 0.6.

Table 4 Illustrative Tabulation of Data for Scoring Net Positives

	Incubation conditions			
Sample	SCDM[b], 30–35°C	SCDM[b], 20–25°C	FTM[c], 30–35°C	Net positives[a]
1	−	−	−	−
2	+	−	−	+
3	+	+	−	+
4	+	+	+	+
5	−	−	−	−
6	+	−	+	+
7	−	−	−	−
8	−	−	+	+
9	−	+	−	+
10	−	−	−	−
Proportion positive	0.40	0.30	0.30	0.60

[a]Positive growth in any one, two, or three of the medium-incubation conditions was scored as a net positive.
[b]SCDM = soybean casein digest medium USP
[c]FTM = fluid thioglycollate medium USP

There are alternative ways of interpreting this data:

(a) When the proportion positive is calculated from each of the individual columns, each individual value is less than 0.6; the value obtained from the net-positive approach must always be higher or equal to that obtained from one medium alone.

(b) Another way of interpreting such data might have been to score each medium as positive or negative and express the total as a proportion of the total number of tests. From this approach a proportion positive of 0.33 would have resulted from the data in Table 4. The proportion positive from the net positive approach must always be higher or equal to the value obtained from this alternative interpretation.

(c) A third way is to give equal weight to each positive and express this as a proportion of the number of samples. In Table 4 the number of samples is ten and the proportion positive calculated by this method would be 1.0 (100%). This method maximizes the value of the proportion positive. It assumes that each medium is absolutely selective for a particular kind of microorganism that is unable to grow in any of the other conditions. It also assumes that contamination of a product item by one kind of microorganism excludes the possibility of contamination by another kind. These assumptions bear no relation to practical circumstances.

The net-positive approach provides a properly conservative means of interpreting multiple media data, and multiple media must be used in the construction of any survival curves that are intended to avoid false negative results from naturally contaminated product items.

2. *Exponential Survival Curves*: Exponential survival curves are linear when the logarithm of the number of survivors (or the surviving fraction, N_t/N_0) is plotted against increasing sterilization treatment on an arithmetic scale. This form of death has been noted for pure culture microbial populations since the beginnings of the twentieth century. It follows the pattern of first-order chemical kinetics and has prompted the assumption that death of microorganisms is the result of some molecule essential for the furtherance of viability having undergone some irreversible reaction.

A simple expression describing exponential survival curves is given in Eq. (2.3):

$$N_t = N_0 \cdot e^{-kt}$$

The practicalities of constructing exponential survival curves are not always straightforward.

(a) Some microorganisms are so sensitive to sterilization treatments that it is impossible to construct any part of the survival curve except for the zero point from colony-count data. Therefore all data must come from quantal response experiments. The number of replicates required to plot a reasonable survival curve may rapidly become limiting.

(b) Some sterilization treatments, particularly heat treatment, are not amenable to precise control of incremental delivery. Heat becomes lethal to microorganisms throughout the time taken to reach the specified sterilizing temperature ("heat-up time") and the time taken to cool down after the specified exposure period.

In research laboratories these difficulties are part of the expected challenge. In industrial control laboratories they are serious distractions from obtaining information quickly, usually the D-value. There are several standard approaches to obtaining D-values from simple quantal response experiments using manageable numbers of replicates and without having to draw out survival curves on semilogarithmic paper. These methods assume exponential survival kinetics and should therefore be used with some caution if there is any doubt.

Probably the most widely known method of calculating D-values from quantal response experiments is the Stumbo [19] method. Each sample should consist of at least ten (and rarely more) replicate items carrying the same number of contaminants (N_0). Samples should be exposed to increments of sterilization treatment, and then each replicate should be tested for viable microorganisms separately in suitable recovery conditions. The number of sterile replicates q is scored after incubation. The D-value may be calculated from

$$D = \frac{t}{\log_{10} N_0 - \log_{10} B} \tag{2.8}$$

where t = duration of sterilization treatment (usually time, but for ionizing radiation t would be dose), N_0 = initial number of microorganisms on each replicate, and $B = 2.3026 \log_{10}(n/q)$, where n is the number of replicates in the sample and q is the number negative (sterile).

A separate D-value is usually calculated for each increment of sub-process sterilization treatment and an overall D-value taken from the arithmetic mean.

The same type of experimental design, allowing that each increment of sub-process sterilization treatment d is equal, may be used to calculate D-values by the Spearman Karber method [20]. The total duration of sterilization treatment should be chosen to cover the whole of the quantal region from t_1, which is defined as the longest time at which every replicate is still found to be nonsterile, to time t_k, which is the shortest exposure at which every replicate is found to be sterile as tested. The Spearman Karber equation allows estimation of a factor u as

$$u = t_k - \frac{d}{2} - \frac{d}{n} \sum_{i=1}^{k-1} r_i \tag{2.9}$$

where u = an estimate of the time of exposure required to inactivate 50% of the replicates, t_k = the shortest time of exposure to yield all sterile replicates, d = the time interval between exposures, n = number of replicates per sample, and $\sum_{i=1}^{k-1} r_i$ = the sum of sterile replicates from t_1, to $(t_k - 1)$.

The D-value can be calculated from u through the expression

$$D = \frac{u}{0.2507 + \log_{10} N_0} \tag{2.10}$$

where N_0 = initial number of microorganisms on each replicate.

Annex 3 illustrates how the Stumbo and Spearman Karber methods can be used to estimate D-values from quantal response results.

3. *"Shouldered" Survival Curves*:   Survival curves that initially show no sensitivity to a sterilization treatment but then respond in a typical exponential manner as exposure continues are referred to as "shouldered." They conform to the mathematical form

$$\frac{N_t}{N_0} = 1 - (1 - e^{-kt})^n \tag{2.11}$$

where all terms are the same as those in Eq. (2.3), plus n, which is called the extrapolation number, i.e., the intercept of the extrapolated exponential portion of the curve onto the N_t/N_0 axis.

They are attributed to one or all of several mechanisms.

(a) Repair. In some microorganisms there may be cellular mechanisms that repair molecular damage done by sterilization treatments. While these mechanisms are operative there will be no loss of viability (the shoulder) until they themselves are irreversibly damaged by the sterilization treatment.

(b) Multitarget concepts acknowledge the likelihood of loss of viability being caused only through more than one essential molecule being irreversibly damaged in the cell.

(c) Multihit concepts acknowledge one vital molecule having to react more than one time before it is permanently lost to its role in the continuance of life.

For the purposes of extrapolating SALs, shouldered survival curves can be treated as exponential curves after making an appropriate allowance for the shoulder. In fact shoulders often become negligible with intense sterilization treatments, for example at high temperatures with saturated steam. However, there is some danger in applying the Stumbo or Spearman Karber methods to shouldered curves. D-values (and therefore the treatment recommended to obtain particular SALs) will be overestimated if the shoulder is not recognized. Whereas this is intrinsically conservative as far as assurance of sterility is concerned, unnecessarily excessive sterilization treatment may have deleterious effects on some other characteristic of a pharmaceutical preparation or medical product.

4. "Tailed" Survival Curves: Tailed survival curves cannot be extrapolated. They are characterized by a slope that diminishes with increasing exposure to the sterilization treatment. They are often described as "concave."

Tailed curves are particularly interesting because they challenge the notion of exponential curves being extrapolated ad infinitum to SALs of 10^{-6}, 10^{-12}, 10^{-18}, etc. How valid is extrapolation if the curve begins to tail off beyond the measurable region?

There is one basic question that ought to be addressed about tailed survival curves: are they artefacts or are they genuine? They have certainly been noted in many experiments. Beside the undoubted occurrence of examples of genetic heterogeneity and heterogeneity of treatment, there are three theories [21] that merit some consideration.

(a) The vitalistic theory has it that individual cells in a population (even a genetically homogeneous population) are not identical; therefore some individuals would be very sensitive to a sterilization treatment, the majority averagely sensitive, and others quite resistant. Although plausible, there is very little evidence to support this concept.

(b) The methods of expression of survival data may create artefactual tails. It has been pointed out by various authors that there is a systematic bias in the Stumbo and other methods of interpreting quantal response data leading to calculated D-values increasing with increasing exposure to sterilization treatment.

(c) The confidence limits of survival curves must be understood to be far broader at longer exposures to sterilization treatments because (whereas the inactivation of a large population of microorganisms is a statistical phenomenon) the death of individual microorganisms at low numbers becomes a series of discrete events [22].

Tails have not been seen throughout the whole range of sterilization treatments. For instance, no genuine case of tailing has been attributed to inactivation by ionizing radiation. This may be because of the nature of biochemical mechanisms of inactivation specific for nucleic acids. On the other hand, it may be attributable to the greater ease and precision with which radiation can be delivered to populations of microorganisms compared with other sterilization treatments. On the other hand, there are many instances reported for heat and chemical methods of sterilization. In a review article on the subject of tails, Cerf [21] concluded that it seems prudent not to ignore the possibility of departures from the exponential order of inactivation of microbial populations if it is desirable to avoid the risk of health or commercial hazards.

5. *Survival Curves with Mixed Cultures*: Although most published survival curves have been obtained in the laboratory using pure cultures of microorganisms, most "real life" sterilization processes must deal with mixed cultures, probably heterogeneously distributed over items. There are comparatively few published data on the behavior of mixed cultures, except as they have arisen by accident as contamination in laboratory studies. There is no reason to believe that the different components within a mixed culture do not act completely independently of one another with respect to their responses to sterilization treatments. This tends to be a fundamental assumption in all approaches to validation of existing sterilization processes and of new process development.

REFERENCES

1. *The Therapeutic Substances Regulations, 1952*. London: Her Majesty's Stationery Office.
2. McKay, A. M. (1992). Viable but non-culturable forms of potentially pathogenic bacteria in water. *Letters in Applied Microbiology* **14**: 129–135.
3. Byrd, J. J., Huai-shu, X., and Colwell, R. R. (1991). Viable but nonculturable bacteria in drinking water. *Applied and Environmental Microbiology* **57**: 875–878.
4. Pearson, A. D., Colwell, R. R., Rollins, D., Watkin-Jones, M., Healing, T., Greenwood, M., Shahamat, M., Jump, E., Hood, M., and Jones, D. M. (1988). Transmission of *C. jejuni* on a poultry farm. In *Campylobacter IV* (B. Kaijser and E. Falsen, eds.). Goteberg, Sweden: University of Goteberg.
5. Sharpe, A. N. (1973). Automation and instrumentation developments for the bacteriology laboratory. In *Sampling—Microbiological Monitoring of Environments* (R. G. Board and D. W. Lovelock, eds.). London: Academic Press.
6. Galante, L. J., Brinkley, M. A., Drennen, J. K., and Lodder, R. A. (1990). Near-infrared spectrometry of microorganisms in liquid pharmaceuticals. *Analytical Chemistry* **62**: 2514–2521.
7. Knudsen, L. F. (1949). Sample size of parenteral solutions for sterility testing. *Journal of the American Pharmaceutical Association* **38**: 332–337.
8. Maxwell Bryce, D. (1956). Tests for the sterility of pharmaceutical preparations. *Journal of Pharmacy and Pharmacology* **8**: 561–572.
9. Tattersal, K. (1961). Control of sterility in a manufacturing process. In *Recent Developments in the Sterilisation of Surgical Materials*. London: Pharmaceutical Press.

10. Brown, M. R. W., and Gilbert, P. (1977). Increasing the probability of sterility of medicinal products. *Journal of Pharmacy and Pharmacology* **29**: 517–523.
11. Canadian Standards Association (1979). Industrial sterilization of medical devices by the steam process, *CSA Standard* Z314.4–M1979. Rexdale, Ontario, Canada: Canadian Standards Association.
12. Doolan, P. T., Dwyer, J., Dwyer, V. M., Fitch, F. R., Halls, N. A., and Tallentire, A. (1985). Towards microbiological quality assurance in radiation sterilization processing: A limiting case model. *Journal of Applied Bacteriology* **58**: 303–306.
13. Bill, A. (1992). Bioburden: Sampling and removal. In *Bioburden in Medical Device and Surgical Dressing Manufacture. Proceedings of EUCOMED Conference, March 23 and 24, 1992*. Brussels, Belgium: EUCOMED.
14. Halls, N. A. (1992). Bioburden: Determination. In *Bioburden in Medical Device and Surgical Dressing Manufacture. Proceedings of EUCOMED Conference, March 23 and 24, 1992*. Brussels, Belgium: EUCOMED.
15. Tallentire, A, Dwyer, J., and Ley, F. J. (1971). Microbiological quality control of sterilized products: Evaluation of a model relating frequency of contaminated items with increasing radiation treatment. *Journal of Applied Bacteriology* **34**: 521–534.
16. Borick, P. M., and Borick, J. A. (1972). Sterility testing of pharmaceuticals, cosmetics and medical devices. In *Quality Control in the Pharmaceutical Industry* (M. S. Cooper, ed.) New York: Academic Press.
17. Doolan, P. T., Halls, N. A., and Tallentire, A. (1988). Sub-process irradiation of naturally contaminated hypodermic needles. *Radiation Chemistry and Physics* **31** (4–6): 669–703.
18. Doolan, P. T., Halls, N. A., Joyce, T. M., and Tallentire, A. (1983). Net positives: Conservative approach to measurement of proportions positive in substerilization process studies. *Applied and Environmental Microbiology* **45** (7): 1283–1285.
19. Stumbo, C. R. (1973). *Thermobacteriology in Food Processing*. 2d ed. New York: Academic Press .
20. Pflug, I. J. (1977). Principles of thermal destruction of microorganisms. In *Disinfection, Sterilization and Preservation*. 2d ed. (S. S. Block, ed.) Philadelphia: Lea and Febiger.
21. Cerf, O. (1977). Tailing of survival curves of bacterial spores. *Journal of Applied Bacteriology* **42**: 1–19.
22. Fredrickson, A. G. (1966). Stochastic models for sterilization. *Biotechnology and Bioengineering* **8**: 167–182.

ANNEX 1. CALCULATING THE PROBABILITIES OF ACCEPTING BATCHES OF PRODUCT BY THE PHARMACOPOEIAL *TEST FOR STERILITY*

The probability of selecting n consecutive sterile items from a population containing a proportion p of nonsterile items is given by the expression

$$(1 - p)^n \qquad\qquad (12.1)$$

The pharmacopoeial *Tests for Sterility* typically pass batches from which twenty items have been tested and shown not to be nonsterile. There is no doubt that it would be unethical to release a batch of product containing nonsterile items in the proportion of one in (say) two hundred.

In this example p would equal 0.005 and n would equal 20. The term

$(1 - p) = 0.995$

Taking logarithms,

$\log_{10} 0.995 = -0.0022$

Solve for $(1 - p)^n$ by multiplying

$20 \times -0.0022 = -0.0435$

Withdrawing from logarithms,

antilog $-0.0435 = 0.9046$

Therefore we would find that even with a frequency of occurrence of one nonsterile item in two hundred, a batch would have a greater than 90% chance of passing the *Test for Sterility*.

ANNEX 2. CALCULATING THE PROBABILITIES OF OCCURRENCE OF STERILE AND NONSTERILE ITEMS IN MULTIITEM EXPERIMENTS

(a) In a multiitem quantal response experiment, 15 items were bulked in each test that could be scored as showing growth or no-growth. Of 20 tests (each of 15 bulked items), one showed growth, i.e., the ratio of nonsterile tests to sterile tests was 0.05.

(b) According to Doolan et al. [17], this ratio is an estimate of the term $(1 - q^n)$.

(c) If $(1 - q^n) = 0.05$, when n is equal to 15, the value of q can be calculated by simplifying terms:

$q^{15} = 0.95$

Taking logarithms,

$\log_{10} 0.95 = -0.0223$

Divide this term by 15 to find $\log_{10} q$; this equals -0.0015, q is therefore the antilogarithm of -0.0015, i.e., 0.997.

(d) The probability of occurrence of a nonsterile item in the population of items from which the sample was drawn can be calculated from $(p + q) = 1$, i.e., p equals 0.003 or one in 333.

ANNEX 3. CALCULATING *D*-VALUES FROM QUANTAL RESPONSE DATA USING THE STUMBO AND SPEARMAN KARBER METHODS

The following data was obtained from a hypothetical investigation into thermal inactivation of bacterial endospores. The initial number of viable spores per replicate was 1×10^6 (N_0).

Time of exposure (min)	Number of replicates (n)	Number sterile (p)
4	10	0
6	10	0
8	10	3
10	10	5
12	10	8
14	10	10

(a) Calculation of *D*-value by the Stumbo method.

$$D = \frac{t}{\log_{10} N_0} - 2.303 \log_{10} \frac{n}{q}$$

where t = time of exposure, N_0 = initial number of microorganisms per replicate, i.e., 10^6, and n/q = number of replicates per sample divided by the number of sterile replicates.

(i)   *D*-value from 6 to 8 min = 2/6 – 3.3 = 0.74 min,
(ii) *D*-value from 6 to 10 min = 4/6 – 2 = 1.0 min
(iii) *D*-value from 6 to 12 min = 6/6 – 1.25 = 1.26 min
(iv) *D*-value from 6 to 14 min = 6/6 – 1 = 1.2 min

Mean *D*-value = 1.05 min.

D-value calculated by the Stumbo method = 1.05 min.

(b) Calculation of *D*-value by the Spearman Karber method.

$$u = t_k - \frac{d}{2} - \frac{d}{n} \sum_{i=1}^{k-1} r_i$$

where t_k = shortest time of exposure for which all replicates were found to be sterile (14 min), d = time increments of exposure (2 min), n = number of repli-cates per sample (15), and $\sum_{i=1}^{k-1} r_i$ = the sum of sterile samples from t_1 to $t_k - 1$

$(0 + 3 + 5 + 8)$, i.e., $u = 14 - 2/2 - 2/10$. $(0 + 3 + 5 + 8) = 9.8$. $D = u/0.2507 + \log_{10}N_0 = 9.8/6.2507$ 1.57 min. D-value calculated by the Spearman Karber method $= 1.57$ min.

3

Sterilization by Gamma Radiation

Terminal sterilization of pharmaceutical dosage forms by ionizing radiation is comparatively rare. On the other hand, ionizing radiation is used extensively for terminal sterilization of heat-sensitive medical devices and for heat-sensitive pharmaceutical packaging components prior to aseptic processing. It is strictly an industrial process; there is no hospital-scale radiation sterilization.

Sterilization by ionizing radiation typically uses gamma rays. There is some use of accelerated electrons, but to a far lesser extent than gamma radia-

53

tion. The pioneering work [1] directed specifically toward evaluating the effectiveness of irradiation as an industrial scale microbicidal process was done in the 1940s. The lethal effects of gamma radiation on microorganisms were already well known, and gamma sources with practical industrial potential were becoming available as by-products of controlled energy release in nuclear reactors. Caesium-137 formed in spent fuel rods was the first isotope considered, but insufficient quantities were available without introducing expensive separation processes. Around the same time, cobalt-59 was beginning to be used as an alternative to steel for neutron absorption in British gas-cooled reactors. Absorption of one neutron per atom converts cobalt-59 to radioactive cobalt-60; separation from other radioactive isotopes was unnecessary. Thus cobalt-60 became the predominant gamma source for industrial sterilization and has remained so despite the U.K. no longer being a significant source of supply.

In the early days of industrial irradiation it was the possibility of food irradiation that excited greatest interest. However, the first commercial application of the microbicidal effects of radiation was sterilization of surgical sutures by Ethicon Inc., Somerville, New Jersey, U.S.A. In the period 1956 to 1964 Ethicon was using a 2 MeV electron beam accelerator to sterilize the greater part of the U.S.A.'s requirement for surgical sutures. The earliest industrial-scale cobalt-60 gamma irradiation plants were opened in 1959 and 1960. The first of these, built to a British design, was opened in Australia in 1959 to eliminate anthrax spores from bales of imported goat hair; the other was built for the United Kingdom Atomic Energy Authority at its Wantage Research Laboratory and was eventually to become allied to the sterilization of medical devices. A caesium-137 plant was opened for Conservatome Industrie, Lyon, France in 1960, also destined to be used for sterilizing medical devices. Progress was somewhat slower in the U.S.A where it was 1963 before the first industrial-scale gamma irradiator was commissioned. Its purpose was to support a food irradiation program which was being initiated by the Quartermaster Corps of the U.S. Army. In 1964 Ethicon replaced their accelerator with a cobalt-60 gamma irradiator.

Medical device sterilization has become the primary application of gamma irradiation, with cobalt-60 remaining the predominant source. Food irradiation is still a controversial subject even in the 1990s. At first, in the 1960s, the rate of expansion of irradiation sterilization was rather slow. The most immediate developments were in Europe, where a single-use medical device industry was developing in pace with the new sterilization technology in a generally favorable regulatory climate. Not so in the U.S.A., where the FDA had initially classified irradiated medical devices as "new drugs" requiring lengthy validation procedures before approval for marketing. This situation had eased by the mid-1970s, partly at least due to growing concern over the probable carcinogenicity of the main alternative "cold" sterilization process with ethylene oxide. In 1975 there were only 55 irradiators in service throughout the world; by 1984 this had doubled to 110, much of this growth being in the U.S.A.

I. RADIATION AND RADIOACTIVITY

All matter is made up of atoms, each atom consisting of a central nucleus circled by negatively charged orbiting electrons. Two types of particle exist within atomic nuclei, positively charged protons and uncharged neutrons. All stable atoms are electrically neutral, the number of protons equalling the number of electrons. Stability is also a function of the number of neutrons in the nucleus because of the balance of forces necessary to bind the nucleus together.

Radioactive materials are materials in which the nuclei of the atoms are unstable. Unstable nuclei are subject to spontaneous decay or disintegration by ejecting a particle in an endeavor to acquire a more stable configuration, thus forming "daughter nuclei." Radiation is emitted as particles are ejected. The SI unit of radioactivity is the becquerel; a radioactive source has an activity of one becquerel if it is disintegrating at a rate of one atom per second.

Consider the stable atom cobalt-59. It has 59 particles in its nucleus. Its atomic number is 27, which means that 27 of the 59 particles are protons; the remaining 32 are neutrons. The purpose for which cobalt-59 was used in the early gas-cooled reactors was to absorb neutrons. When cobalt-59 is bombarded by neutrons, an extra neutron is added to the nucleus, thus forming the unstable radioactive isotope cobalt-60. Radioactive decay of cobalt-60 is a single-stage process to stabilize to its daughter, nickel-60, with emission of one gamma ray photon (a pulse of electromagnetic energy of extremely short wavelength and high energy) and one beta particle (a rapidly moving electron).

Radioactive isotopes emit different types of radiation:

(a) Alpha particles. An alpha particle consists of two protons and two neutrons. When alpha particles pass through materials, they knock off electrons from nearby atoms, gradually slowing down and losing energy as they do so. Even very energetic alpha particles are brought to rest in a few centimeters of air. Alpha decay of an isotope may, however, also produce a release of gamma radiation (see below).

(b) Beta particles. A beta particle is a high-velocity electron that loses its energy in the same way as an alpha particle. It is capable of penetrating far further through materials than alpha particles, for instance up to a few inches of aluminum. This type of radiation is sometimes used for sterilization, usually from electron accelerators rather than from radioactive isotopes, but it imposes quite severe practical limitations on the depth of product that can be presented to the source. This is not because microbiological contaminants need to be killed within the depth of a material (they are usually a surface contamination) but because sterilants are required to penetrate through packaging materials and to surfaces that may be obscured by other depths of materials.

(c) Gamma rays. Gamma rays are photons of electromagnetic radiation with energies in the range of 1 keV to 10 MeV. They are very similar to x-rays. They are very penetrative through matter. They only lose energy when they collide with a nucleus, but they lose all their energy in one collision. Thus gamma rays are able to pass through matter with the same energy as they had when they entered, just fewer of them emerge. Some always penetrate any thickness of a barrier, but the numbers get fewer and fewer with thickness. This property of penetration is the first and most important property of gamma radiation as a robust process for industrial sterilization.

As time goes by, the activity of all radioactive sources diminishes according to an exponential law characterized by its half-life. The half-life is the time taken for the activity to fall to half of its original value. Cobalt-60 has a half-life of 5.3 years; caesium-137 has a half-life of 30 years. Thus a radioactive isotope is decaying and losing activity at all times regardless of whether it is being used or not. This factor has economic implications for industrial-scale irradiation.

The alternative to isotope sources of radiation is the production of accelerated electrons. Accelerators have an economic advantage over isotopes in that they can be switched off when not required. Their disadvantage is in their poor penetrative properties.

An accelerator is a device in which an electric field is developed by application of a voltage at opposite ends of a linear path. The greater the voltage, the faster the speed of the electrons; the faster the speed of the electrons, the greater their penetrative power through matter. For practical sterilization purposes, accelerators of less than 100 MeV are being used for products such as hypodermic needles in which the requirement for penetration is minimal.

II. EFFECTS OF RADIATION ON MICROORGANISMS

Radiation damage to biological systems and other materials is caused by the energy absorbed from the radiation. The damage is proportional to the amount of energy absorbed. The amount of energy absorbed is referred to as dose (correctly, absorbed dose), and it is measured in units of energy per kilogram. The SI unit of dose is the gray (Gy), which is defined as an absorbed radiation dose of one joule per kilogram. Where time of sterilization treatment was referred to in Chapter 2, dose should be substituted when dealing with irradiation.

Prior to the introduction of SI units, the unit of absorbed dose of radiation was the rad (also krad and Mrad), and this unit still appears in some compendia, regulatory documents, and other sources of information. For reference, 100 rad is equivalent to one gray, and 2.5 Mrad is equivalent to 25 kGy.

A. Molecular and Cellular Effects of Radiation

The absorption of ionizing radiation in matter leads to numerous phenomena of high complexity. In biological materials these can be categorized within four stages:

(a) A physical stage in which extremely unstable excited or ionized molecules (primary products) are produced from interaction of gamma ray photons with orbiting electrons.

(b) A physicochemical stage in which the primary products react spontaneously or in collision with each other, bonds are broken, and highly reactive ions, radicals, and trapped charges are formed. It is the reaction of these reactive groups that produces observed changes.

(c) A chemical stage. This is the reaction and interaction of the reactive groups described in (b) above. It is basically a stage of achieving thermal equilibrium.

(d) The biological stage comprising a series of biochemical reactions at different levels of cellular organization, giving rise to observable biological effects. Loss of viability of the microbial cell is principally due to dimerization of DNA bases and scission and cross-linking of the sugar-phosphate backbone of DNA.

Microorganisms of a given type may respond differently to radiation according to different physical or chemical conditions existing within the cell or in its immediate environment. Of these environmental factors, the most extensively studied have been the effects of oxygen and the effects of hydration.

Microorganisms are more sensitive to radiation when oxygen is present during and after irradiation than in environments from which oxygen has been excluded. In other words, oxygen sensitizes microorganisms to radiation. This is likely due to reaction of oxygen with free radicals formed by ionization of target molecules. One hypothesis postulates radiation giving rise to two types of damaged molecule, R' and R". The first of these is a free radical without effect on the survival of cells unless oxygen reacts with it:

$R \rightsquigarrow R' + H^+ + e^-$ nonlethal

$R' + O_2 \rightarrow RO_2$ lethal

The second type of damaged molecule is lethal irrespective of the presence or absence of oxygen:

R $\Lambda\Lambda\Lambda$R"   lethal

Whereas oxygen sensitizes microorganisms, water (in the presence of oxygen) protects microorganisms from radiation damage. The drier cells are, the more sensitive they are to radiation-induced lethal damage. The reason for this has to do with irradiation damage that occurs only when cells are irradiated in the presence of oxygen (the immediate oxygen effect). This effect is believed to be due to interaction of oxygen with extremely short-lived species produced at the time of irradiation. Increasing cellular water content results in a substantial decrease in this type of damage, presumably due to competition from the water molecules for these short-lived radicals.

B. Effects of Radiation on Microbial Populations

In a typical experiment designed for quantitative study of irradiation inactivation of microorganisms, a population of cells is exposed to a series of incremental doses of radiation. After each dose the numbers of microorganisms surviving are counted and plotted as fractions of the original population on a logarithmic scale against radiation dose on an arithmetic scale. Radiation inactivation of microbial populations is probably the best researched of any microbicidal treatment. This is primarily because of the precision with which doses of radiation can be delivered to microbial populations. Radiation experiments do not have to introduce compensatory factors for heat-up and cool-down in the way that thermal inactivation studies must, nor are there any residues or traces of radiation left behind when the sample is removed from the radiation field. A secondary but highly significant factor is the comparability of radiation results. An absorbed dose of x Gy has the same significance wherever it is delivered, and for whatever configuration the sample was irradiated in. There are no local differences caused by equipment design or irregularity, as long as the measurement of dose is done correctly. Importantly, the rate of delivery of dose (dose rate) has no effect on the radiation response of microbial populations.

Survival curves for irradiated pure cultures of microbial populations conform to the idealized types described in Chapter 2. In radiation microbiology the D-value is invariably called the D_{10} value. It is doubtful whether a truly "tailed" survival curve has ever been seen in a properly conducted irradiation study of pure cultures. There are, however, major differences seen from microorganism to microorganism and from condition to condition.

The extent to which various microorganisms respond to radiation is very much determined by different abilities to "repair" radiation-induced damage. Differences in these abilities give microorganisms unique innate sensitivities to radiation, as was shown by Tallentire [2] when five different types of microor-

Table 1 Innate Sensitivity of Microorganisms to Gamma Radiation when Grown Under Similar Conditions and Irradiated Under Identical Conditions

Organism	Shape of curve	D_{10} (Gy)
Ps. aeruginosa	Exponential	20
Staph. aureus	Exponential	100
Strep. faecium	Shouldered	500
B. pumilus spores	Exponential	1700
B. sphaericus spores	Exponential	4600

Source: Tallentire (1980)

ganism showed appreciably different response to radiation (Table 1) when grown under as near identical conditions as possible and irradiated under exactly the same conditions.

The limits of innate sensitivity are wide, typified by D_{10} values of around 20 Gy for *Pseudomonas* spp up to 4.6 kGy for spores of *Bacillus sphaericus* when irradiated in air. Typically, gram-negative bacteria are more sensitive to radiation than gram-positive bacteria, and gram-positive bacteria are more sensitive than bacterial endospores. Danish workers have isolated some unusual gram-positive cocci identified with *Streptococcus faecium* A2 and *Micrococcus radiodurans,* which are exceedingly resistant to radiation owing to extended "shouldered" inactivation curves.

The effects of oxygen and water described above as affecting radiation damage at the cellular level are reflected in the responses of microbial populations to radiation. Other chemical factors may also protect or sensitize microorganisms. The effects of temperature on radiation response of microbial populations tend to be complex, but in general, increases in temperature during irradiation bring about slight increases in radiation sensitivity. These effects may be complicated by the presence or absence of oxygen and water.

III. APPLICATIONS

The most time-proven methods of sterilization have been the use of high temperatures and filtration. However, medical practice has always included objects that are neither filterable nor able to withstand high temperatures, which were "sterilized" by methods of doubtful effectiveness, such as liquid sterilizing fluids or formalin cabinets. In the 1940s and 1950s this problem began to be aggravated by rapid advances in surgery and anaesthetics, which demanded the use of heat-sensitive plastic tubing, valves, and prostheses. The outcome of these changes was the provision of as many as possible of the cheaper plastic and rubber items as single-use disposable products presterilized by the manufacturer within individual sealed packs. This promoted the introduction of "cold" sterilization methods, mainly gamma irradiation and exposure to ethylene oxide, which are only practical on an industrial scale. The adoption of cold sterilized single-use medical devices also obviated many of the risks and costs to hospitals that arise from cleaning and resterilizing complex devices.

The highest product temperatures reached in industrial-scale gamma irradiators is usually in the range 30–40°C depending on source strength. Many devices or components made from plastics deform at thermal sterilization temperatures but are quite capable of withstanding the temperatures reached in gamma irradiation. For reference, the Vicat softening points (the maximum temperature to which a polymeric component may be subjected without deforming) of some commercially available plastics suitable for medical applications are given in Table 2. As early as 1964 the range of medical products being sterilized by exposure to gamma radiation extended to plastic disposable hypodermic syringes and needles, surgical blades, plastic and rubber catheters, drainage bags, blood lancets, cannulae, diaysis units, infusion sets, gauze and cotton wool dressings, and surgeon's rubber gloves. Within the pharmaceutical industry the pharmacopoeias acknowledge gamma irradiation as a sterilization process applicable to drug substances and final dosage forms, but its main application is sterilization of heat-sensitive containers for aseptic filling processes. The

Table 2 Vicat Softening Temperatures of Radiation-Sterilizable Medical Grade Molding Polymers

Polymer	Brand name	Manufacturer	Vicat softening temperature (°C)
LDPE	Resin 722	Dow Chemical, Midland, Michigan, U.S.A.	90
HDPE	290 B1	Amoco Chemicals Corp., Chicago, Illinois, U.S.A.	125
Polypropylene	Tenite	Eastman Chemical Products, Kingsport, Tennessee, U.S.A.	143
ABS	Cycolac DH	Borg Warner, Amsterdam, The Netherlands	97
PVC	Alpha 3006R-82 Clear	Alpha Chemicals, 40 Parham Drive, Eastleigh, Hampshire, 505 4NU, England	75

various effects of gamma radiation on specific pharmaceuticals were reviewed by Jacobs in 1985 [3], but few general conclusions could be drawn except that solid preparations are generally more stable than liquids, and frozen solutions are more stable than liquids.

Theoretically, it is unlikely that aqueous pharmaceutical formulations are going to be amenable to radiation sterilization. Consider the drug *ranitidine* (molecular weight of 314) in 1% aqueous solution:

The number of drug molecules per gram molecule (314 g) is equal to 6×10^{23} (Avogadro's number).

Therefore 100 g of solution would contain 1 g of ranitidine or approximately 2×10^{21} molecules.

Therefore 1 g of aqueous preparation would contain 2×10^{19} molecules.

On irradiation, the greater part of the energy would be deposited in the water to form reactive species; essentially none of the energy would be deposited in the drug.

The yield of reactive species, from water can be calculated from the energy equivalent (1 kGy is equal to 6.242×10^{18} eV/g) and the radiation chemical yield G (the mean number of elementary entities produced, destroyed, or changed per 100 eV) for water (equal to 3). For 25 kGy the yield of reactive species from water is equal to 4.5×10^{18} per g.

The proportion of molecules of ranitidine in 1% aqueous preparation that would be changed as a result of irradiation at 25 kGy is calculable on the basis of a chemical change occurring on every encounter between drug molecule and reactive species, thus

$$\frac{4.5 \times 10^{18}}{2 \times 10^{19}} \times 100 = 22.5\%$$

On the other hand, irradiation could theoretically do less damage to the same drug in its solid form, thus

1 g of ranitidine contains 2×10^{21} molecules.

The electron volt (eV) equivalent of 25 kGy is calculable from 1 kGy being equivalent to 6.242×10^{18} eV/g, to equal 1.5×10^{20} eV/g.

Each primary ionization requires 30 eV.

Therefore 25 kGy would induce ($1.5 \times 10^{20}/30$) or 5×10^{18} ionizations per g.

The proportion of molecules of ranitidine in solid form changed as a result of irradiation at 25 kGy is calculable on the basis of each primary ionization producing a chemical change, thus $(5 \times 10^{18}/2 \times 10^{21}) \times 100 = 0.25\%$

On the cautionary side it was noted that it is usually not possible to predict the radiation stability of pharmaceutically active substances from previous knowledge of other related substances, as minor differences in chemical structure can apparently have significant bearing on radiation stability and on therapeutic activity.

Compared with all other methods of sterilization (hot or cold), gamma radiation has the overwhelming advantage of penetration through materials. The advantages of penetration extend through all aspects of medical products, from initial design to the final presentation of the products in their shipping packs. Nature abhors sterility; a sterile environment, whether a microbiological culture medium or a medical device, can only be maintained sterile if separated from the nonsterile world by barriers that are impermeable to microorganisms. For terminal sterilization, these barriers must be designed with the consideration that the sterilant must penetrate to all parts of the device that might come into contact with the patient either directly or indirectly through a delivered therapeutic agent. This is a major constraint upon all industrial-scale sterilization processes except gamma irradiation. Some particular situations where this is a decided advantage are considered below.

(a) Internal cavities. Many devices have sealed internal cavities; for instance, syringe plungers are usually fitted with elastomeric tips that seal with an interference fit to the barrel wall at two or three diameters separated by one or two internal cavities. A similar situation applies where manufacturers only cap or seal the fluid paths of devices for which the sterility of the internal lumina (e.g., infusion sets, catheters, etc.) needs to be guaranteed. If steam or ethylene oxide is the chosen method of sterilization, special provisions must be made for complete replacement of air by the sterilant from these internal cavities. This may frequently require recourse to methods and design considerations that introduce other compromises and conflicts, for instance, acceptance of higher sterilization temperatures than necessary or introduction of vented caps fitted with microbial filters or tortuous paths.

(b) Selection of packaging materials. Permeable materials are necessary for unit containers subjected to ethylene oxide sterilization or steam sterilization (unless the contents of the container are liquid). Paper is widely used for devices and surgical products because of its permeability. However, it is opaque, it tears easily on devices with sharp edges, and it is not always impermeable to microorganisms. Alternative permeable materials, such as spun-bonded polyolefins (Tyvek) are very expensive. The effectiveness of penetration of gamma radiation has allowed the introduction of numerous nonpermeable polymeric packaging materials to the manufacture of unit containers; their advantages over traditional materials include transparency, durability, and cost effectiveness. Furthermore, with gamma irradiation, seals are not subjected to potentially deleterious effects of moisture and pressure changes seen in other methods of sterilization.

Another advantage of gamma radiation over other terminal sterilization processes is its reliability. The lethality of gamma radiation is dependent solely on dose. It is self-evident that controlling one parameter must be simpler than control of any interaction of two or more parameters, and that processes that are easily controlled are inherently more reliable than those that are not.

The greatest disadvantage to gamma irradiation of plastic medical devices and pharmaceutical containers is the deleterious effects that radiation has on some polymers that might otherwise be preferred materials of manufacture. When radiation excites or ionizes the atoms or subunits of polymeric materials, the two principal effects are chain scission and cross-linking. Chain scission randomly ruptures the bonds that link the monomeric subunits of the macromolecule. On its own it reduces chain length and leads to gas evolution and unsaturation. When it is accompanied by cross-linking between the resulting low molecular weight fragments, the end results are crystalline structures and three-dimensional matrices within the polymer.

These effects are dose dependent and differ from one polymer to another according to their molecular structure. Polymers containing aromatic groups are more resistant to radiation-induced chain scission and cross-linking than purely aliphatic molecules. However, predictability is further complicated by commercially available polymers being only very rarely pure macromolecules; usually there are other compounds included in their formulations, e.g., antioxidants, light-stabilizers, plasticizers, and fillers. Some of these, included as processing aids, may exacerbate radiation damage; others may have the opposite effect and improve radiation stability or disguise its deleterious effects. Some grades of polymer are specifically claimed to be radiation stable. From an end-use point of view, the most serious adverse effects of these interactions of radiation with polymeric materials are discoloration and weakened mechanical properties. In medical devices markets, white and blue are perceived as "clean" colors, yellow and brown as "dirty" colors; radiation-induced discoloration in susceptible polymers ranges from slight yellowing to complete opacity. The induction of brittleness and fragility in products intended to have strength and resilience are the most damaging effects of radiation on mechanical properties.

These issues have not prevented a whole array of polymers becoming available for the manufacture of medical devices sterilizable within the dose ranges usually recommended (Table 3). The two principal polymers that have

Table 3 Examples of Polymers Used for Irradiation-Sterilized Medical Devices

Polymer	Application examples	Processing	Stability up to 25 kGy	Stability > 25 kGy	Comments
ABS - Acrylonitrile Butadiene Styrene	Closure-piercing devices, roller clamps	Injection Molding	Good	To 1000 kGy	Rigid, most often trans-lucent/opaque
Acrylics	Luer connectors, injection-sites	Injection Molding	Good	To 1000 kGy	Clear with slight yellow-ness after irradiation
Cellulosics	Ventilation filters	Various	Good	To 200 kGy	Repeated irradiation embrittles
Fluoroplastics	Tubing	Extrusion	—[a]	—[a]	PTFE unstable, to FEP stable at 25 kGy and higher
Polyamides (Nylon)	Fluid filters	Extrusion	Good	To 500 kGy	May harden on irradiation
Polyethylene	Protector caps	Injection molding	Good	To 1000 kGy	Translucent/opaque, soft/waxy feel
Polypropylene	Hypodermic syringes	Injection molding	—[a]	—[a]	Embrittles over time
Polystyrene	Syringe plungers	Injection molding	Good	To 10,000 kGy	Rigid
Polyvinyl chloride	Tubing, drip chambers	Injection molding extrusion	—[a]	—[a]	Discolors
PAN - Polystyrene Acrylonitrile	Hypodermic syringes	Injection molding	Good	To 5000 kGy	Rigid, clear

[a]Specific to a particular formulation.

proved problematic with regard to radiation stability are polypropylene and polyvinyl chloride (PVC).

(a) Polypropylene is in many respects an ideal material for manufacture of medical devices. It is biologically inert, naturally translucent, resilient, and flexible. From a manufacturing point of view it can be processed by blow-molding or injection-molding, and molded parts exhibit only minor shrinkage and accept print fairly readily.

Polypropylene is the most widely used material for the manufacture of sterile disposable hypodermic syringes. However, the suitability of irradiation sterilization for polypropylene devices was until the 1980s severely restricted by yellowing and insidious embrittlement after irradiation.

Radiation-induced discoloration of polypropylene is due mainly to the formation of colored radiolysis by-products from phenolic compounds included as processing aids in commercially available formulations. Embrittlement is initiated through chain scission bringing about the reaction

$$R\text{-}R \xrightarrow{} R\cdot + R$$

which continues in the presence of oxygen over time:

$$R\cdot + O_2 \rightarrow RO_2\cdot$$

$$RO_2\cdot + RH \rightarrow ROOH + R\cdot$$

$$RO_2\cdot + R\cdot \rightarrow ROOR$$

$$RO_2\cdot + RO_2\cdot \rightarrow ROOR + O_2$$

$$R\cdot + R\cdot \rightarrow R\text{-}R$$

In polypropylene this process of autooxidation is long-lived, leading eventually to severe embrittlement, which may render a formulation that could have appeared to be acceptable (when assessed immediately after irradiation) totally unacceptable a few months later.

Both yellowing and embrittlement of polypropylene are dose dependent but are significant at or around 25 kGy (the customary compendial dose for sterilizing medical devices). The extent of radiation-induced discoloration can be relieved by use of phosphite stabilizers. Stability against embrittlement may be improved by adding antioxidants, but these may in turn create problems such as surface "blooms."

An alternative approach to improving radiation stability has been through coupling the desirable processing properties of polypropylene with the radiation stability of polyethylene to form copolymers (polyallomers). Block polymers in which the chains comprise polymerized segments of each of the monomers are as amenable to processing as polypropylene while having better clarity and radiation stability.

(b) PVC has a wide variety of applications and potential applications as a material of manufacture for medical devices and packaging films. It is

clear and transparent and may be flexible or rigid according to its plasti-
cizer content. It is widely used in the form of extruded tubing for infusion
sets, catheters, etc. Deleterious mechanical effects are not generally seen
at sterilizing doses of radiation, but special formulations are necessary if
severe discoloration is to be avoided. Discoloration is initiated by radiation-induced free-radical formation, usually by scission of the carbon-chlo-
rine bond of the PVC:

$$\sim CH - CHCl \rightarrow CH_2 - CH\cdot + Cl\cdot$$

The free-radical reacts with the PVC chain at a methylene hydrogen atom
to form conjugated double bonds within the PVC chain:

$$\sim CH_2 - CHCl + Cl\cdot \rightarrow \sim CH = CH\sim + HCl$$

The polyenes formed in these reactions cause discoloration through their
absorption in the UV and visible spectra. Conventional formulations of
PVC become perceptibly yellow at 5 kGy and deep brown at 25 kGy.
Radiation-stable formulations of PVC usually incorporate free radical
scavengers to compensate for the reactivity but often still require the inclusion of optical brighteners or blue tints to disguise the discoloration.

Finally, gamma irradiation sterilized products are safe products. Gamma
radiation leaves no residues, and at doses used for sterilization it does not have
sufficient energy to induce radioactivity in materials it traverses. Furthermore,
gamma irradiation does not pose a radioactive waste problem. The radioactive
material is completely contained, and when sources become too weak for industrial purposes there are contractual agreements to ensure their return to their
source of supply, where they may either be disposed of or resold for installation
in research irradiators.

IV. INDUSTRIAL-SCALE COBALT-60 GAMMA IRRADIATION
STERILIZATION

A dose of 25 kGy (2.5 Mrad) is quoted in all of the major pharmacopoeias as
suitable for sterilizing medical products. This dose is also quoted in the *Guide to
Good Manufacturing Practice for Medical Devices and Surgical Products,* 1981
[4]. This document emphasises the need for the process specification to be
accompanied by high standards of GMP in the manufacture of the product prior
to irradiation. The USP elaborates on the potential for 25 kGy to have damaging
effects on some products and is prepared to accept properly validated lower
doses that achieve SALs of 10^{-6}.

From the very early days of irradiation sterilization, the major regulatory
bodies have not demanded pharmacopoeial sterility testing of irradiated finished
products. This has been an endorsement of the effectiveness and the levels of

control achievable in industrial-scale irradiators. At the international level there is virtually universal agreement regarding standards of plant layout, construction and operation; measurement and monitoring of dose; assignment of responsibility; and other physical aspects of the technology. The whole basis of successful industrial-scale irradiation sterilization lies in the fact that its technology imposes certain obligatory safety measures, interlocks, fail-safe devices, back-up systems, etc., that in turn make it difficult for dose delivery to be compromised by either mechanical or human error.

A. Cobalt-60 Gamma Irradiators

1. Shielding: No two industrial-scale cobalt-60 gamma irradiators are identical, but all share certain similarities arising from having been designed around a need to have products exposed to radiation while at the same time preventing escape of radiation to the outside world. It is quite usual for the "shielding" to be the most striking feature of gamma irradiation plants. In a typical plant (Fig. 1), irradiation takes place within a building (the "cell") which has its roof and walls built from poured concrete 2 m thick. This allows safe use of source

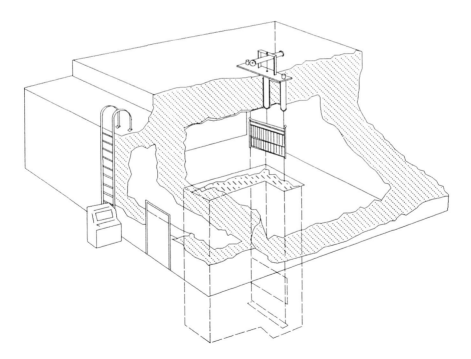

Fig. 1 Simplified representation of a cobalt-60 gamma irradiator.

strengths of up to 0.75×10^{17} to 1.5×10^{17} becquerels of cobalt-60 (two to three million curies [Ci]).

Such massive shielding is necessary because there is no definite range to penetration of gamma radiation through matter. For passage through any particular material the number of gamma ray photons diminishes in an exponential manner until they become insignificant compared to environmental background radiation. This attenuation of gamma radiation as a result of passage through an absorbing material can be described by the equation

$$I_t = I_0^{-ut} \tag{3.1}$$

where I_t = the intensity of irradiation after passing through a barrier of thickness t; I_0 = the intensity of irradiation if the barrier had not been present; and u = a constant, the linear absorption coefficient of the material comprising the barrier.

The linear absorption coefficient u is a function of the type of material and of the energy of the incident photons. Gamma radiation from cobalt-60 is more penetrating than gamma radiation from caesium-137, and so different thicknesses of the same material are required to obtain identical levels of shielding. Equation (3.1) is most commonly used to calculate the thickness required from shielding materials to attenuate radiation to one half (the half value layer, HVL) or one tenth (the tenth value layer, TVL) of its intensity. Because attenuation is an exponential function, the HVL and TVL are independent of the intensity of radiation for which shielding is required. Some HVLs and TVLs for gamma radiation and typical shielding materials are shown in Table 4. According to these figures, the concrete walls 2 m thick of industrial-scale cobalt-60 gamma irradiators should reduce the intensity of irradiation by a factor of about 10^{10}; the same degree of attenuation should be obtainable with about 6 m of water or 360 mm of lead.

Table 4 Approximate Half Value Layers (HVL) and Tenth Value Layers (TVL) of Shielding Materials Used in Large-Scale Gamma Irradiators

Shielding material	Shielding thickness (mm)			
	Caesium-137		Cobalt-60	
	HVL	TVL	HVL	TVL
Lead	7	22	12	40
Steel	16	53	21	70
Concrete	48	157	62	200
Water	150	540	200	700

2. The Source: The world's largest producer of cobalt-60 is Nordion, formerly Atomic Energy of Canada Ltd., Kanata, Ontario, Canada. The starting material is nickel-plated slugs of chemically pure cobalt-59 sealed into zircalloy capsules using a tungsten-inert gas welding process. These primary capsules are held in a nuclear reactor as neutron absorbers for one year or longer in order to reach the required radioactive strength of cobalt-60. The radioactive capsules are then removed from the reactor and double-encapsulated into stainless steel "pencils" about 11 mm in diameter by 450 mm long.

In most Nordion irradiators the pencils of cobalt-60 are mounted vertically in a source rack. The configuration is formally described as laminar. The source rack is suspended from a hoist mechanism on the roof of the cell such that it is movable between two locations. One of these locations is in the center of the cell in a position where product can be moved around the source during its irradiation. The other location is below floor level. This is for safe storage of the source when product irradiation needs to be interrupted for loading or maintenance work within the cell.

Irradiators may be of "wet" storage or "dry" storage types. In Nordion plants the storage location for the source rack is typically at the bottom of a pool of water 6 m deep sunk in the cell floor. For dry storage, a pit is provided in the cell floor and the source rack is fixed to a shielding plug that fills the mouth of the pit when the source rack has been lowered into the storage location. Dry storage pits may be less than 2 m deep with the plug amounting to more than half of the depth. The majority of modern irradiators are of the wet storage type, but each method has its own advantages and disadvantages. Geological conditions may favor dry storage in the event of the substratum being unsuitable for deep excavation. On the other hand, with wet storage the source rack is visible through the water. This makes it possible to inspect, manipulate, and if necessary correct problems *in situ*.

For source loadings in excess of about 2×10^{16} becquerels (500 kCi) both types of storage are likely to require cooling. A heat output of 1 kW can be expected from 2.5×10^{16} becquerels of cobalt-60. For wet storage, cooling usually consists of external circulation of the pool water through a chiller; for dry storage, there may be a need for cooling pipes to be incorporated into the concrete shielding around the pit. Wet Storage cooling water must be maintained ion-free to prevent corrosion of the stainless steel pencils.

3. Conveyors: There must always be some mechanism within industrial gamma irradiators for moving product around the source and in and out of the cell. On the basis of the type of conveyor used, gamma irradiators may be designed for continuous or batch operation.

Most modern irradiators are of the continuous type with open loop conveyor systems that allow the product to be loaded and unloaded outside the cell without interrupting the process. Entry and exit of the product is usually via a double-walled concrete passage incorporating right angle bends—the maze. Each of the two walls of the maze is usually about half as thick as the roof and the other walls, such that together they offer the same attenuation as other parts of the shielding. The right angle bends and the length of the maze prevent radiation from escaping to the outside world, because radiation, like light, travels in straight lines. The dose delivered to the product is controlled via the speed of the conveyor; at slow speeds a particular product would be exposed to the source for a longer time and therefore receive a higher dose of radiation than it would if the conveyor were moving the product at a faster speed.

Batch irradiators are far rarer; conveyors are of the closed loop type wholly contained within the cell. Loading is done by personnel who enter the cell with the source in its safe storage location. The source is then brought to its operational position in the center of the cell and the conveyor is set in motion, moving the product around the source. When sufficient time has elapsed to ensure that the product has absorbed its appropriate dose, the source rack is returned to its safe location, and personnel enter the cell to unload and reload the conveyor.

There are broadly two types of product handling conveyors used in cobalt-60 gamma irradiators, conveyor bed designs and carrier designs.

In conveyor bed systems the product is packed into tote boxes, termed irradiation containers. These are supported from beneath by rollers or trays along which the containers are transported into the irradiator, past the source, and back out again. Figure 2 shows the Nordion JS 8500 continuous-type gamma irradiator. In this sterilizer the irradiation container is an aluminum tote box approximately 900 mm high, 600 mm in length, and 400 mm in depth. The 400 mm dimension separates the two sides of the tote, which alternately face the incident radiation as the container is moved from one stretch of the conveyor to the next.

The conveyor has two vertical product levels and two passes on each side of the source. The containers are indexed through 63 positions by discharge of eight pneumatic cylinders (one at each end of each stretch of the conveyor), assisted by cross-transfer cylinders that move the product between parallel stretches and an elevator that moves the product one container at a time from the bottom to the top level. Some operators of this type of irradiator have achieved an economy by substituting cardboard shippers for aluminum totes as irradiation containers. The economy is from the manning required for one loading operation instead of two loading and one unloading operations. The cost can be in increased downtime if the purchased cardboard shippers do not meet the same close dimensional tolerances of the aluminum totes. A small dimensional or geometric irregularity magnified through a line of eight totes may too easily cause conveyor jams and increased downtime.

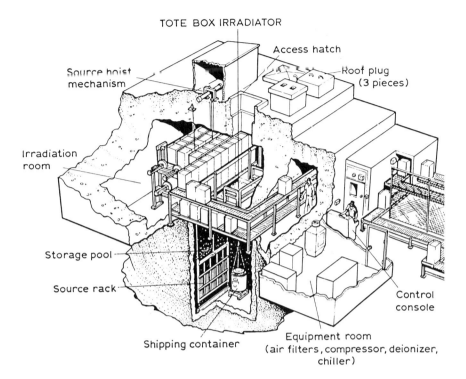

Fig. 2 Nordion JS 8500 continuous-type gamma irradiator.

In carrier-type irradiators, product packages are moved around the source in aluminum carriers suspended from an overhead monorail. One such irradiator is Nordion's JS 8900 (Fig. 3), which has a 3 m high carrier and can be built with two, three, or four passes on each side of the source. The source rack is termed an "overlapping source" because it is 4 m high versus the 3 m carrier. Product is loaded outside the cell, one circuit of the track is completed, and then the carriers are unloaded and reloaded with new product for sterilization.

Some carrier-type irradiators have shelved carriers taller than the source rack. These are called "overlapping product" irradiators. This design is comparatively unusual in newer irradiators. Movement of the product from shelf to shelf within the carriers is needed to achieve reasonable levels of dose uniformity. Each product package is loaded onto the lowest shelf of a container; it moves through the cell showing opposite faces to the incident radiation as it passes down each stretch of the conveyor. On completion of a complete passage on the bottom shelf, the product box is transferred automatically to the second shelf by means of an elevator and a pneumatic ram situated outside the cell.

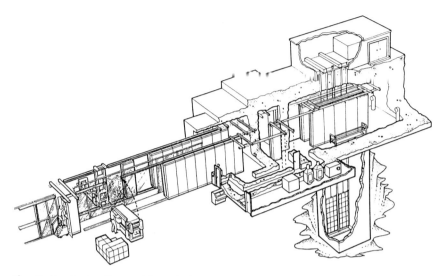

Fig. 3 Carrier irradiator with vertical and horizontal load/unload positions.

Each product box makes four complete transits through the irradiator starting on the lowest and finishing on the highest shelf.

B. Control of Dose

The lethality of gamma radiation is dependent solely on one parameter— absorbed dose. In practice, absorbed dose is dependent upon the strength of the source, the apparent density (bulk density) of the product packages being irradiated, and the time of exposure. There is no fundamental relationship between source strength and dose absorbed in medical products; an empirical relationship must be determined for particular irradiators and products by means of measurement of dose (dosimetry). This is the key work that must be done in validating a particular irradiation sterilization process. It addresses the question of how long a particular product should be exposed in a particular irradiation container to a source of a particular strength to have absorbed a specified minimum dose in all parts of the container.

1. Validation by Dose-Mapping: All variable conditions must be specified during validation and controlled in routine practice thereafter. A loading pattern must be established for each type of product. This should specify the number, position, and orientation of product packages within the irradiation container. The distribution of density within the loading pattern should be chosen to be as near uniform as possible in order to minimize dose variations.

The so-called bulk density of the irradiation container is an important control parameter in irradiation. This is the gross weight of the loaded irradiation container divided by its volume. It is used as the main criterion for deciding whether two product types may be irradiated one after the other in a continuous-type irradiator without overdosing one or underdosing the other. Since the volume of the irradiation container is dictated by the dimensions of the conveyor, many operators are content to monitor the weight of loaded containers for this purpose.

Following the establishment of a loading pattern, a dose mapping exercise should be done. A loaded irradiation container should have a large number of dosimeters distributed to a defined pattern throughout its volume. The container should then be passed through the irradiator, noting the date, the time of exposure to the source, and the speed of travel of the conveyor. At all times when the "dose mapping container" is in the irradiator, the other containers filling the conveyor should be of the same bulk density as the investigational material. It is normal to do dose mappings in triplicate containers to account for any unexpected variation. It is a matter of choice whether they are run adjacent to one another.

The purposes of dose mapping are

(a) To determine dose uniformity. The ratio of the highest dose to the lowest dose (the max/min ratio) can be of importance to successful irradiation of materials that may be adversely affected by high doses of radiation. It is important that the specified sterilizing dose is understood to be a minimum dose, in other words, product in the low dose zone should receive no less than the specified sterilization dose; all other parts of the container are therefore overdosed in relation to this product and to the specified dose.

(b) To determine the low dose point or zone. This is the significant point or zone in the container as far as sterilization is concerned. All parts of the product being sterilized must receive the specified sterilizing dose as a minimum. Routine dosimeters need not be placed in the low dose zone, indeed it may be wholly impractical, but the relationship of the routine dosimeter location to the low dose zone must be known.

(c) To determine the appropriate conveyor speed (exposure time) for the specified sterilizing dose. With some prior knowledge it is usually possible for a dose mapping to serve the purpose of confirming a conveyor speed predetermined to be appropriate to the specified sterilizing dose.

Dose mapping validations are necessary for new products, new irradiation container loading patterns, altered conveyor configurations, and changes to the source, including source replenishments.

2. Routine Dose Control: Routine dose control is straightforward as long as reliable validation–dose mapping information is available. The conveyor speed that assures a dose of *x* kGy on a particular date need only be adjusted to compensate for source decay, and thereafter the required dose will always be delivered and received. Cobalt-60 decays exponentially with a half-life of 5.3 years; for practical purposes this means that the conveyor speed should be slowed down by 1% per month to ensure that a particular product continues to receive a specified dose over time.

Irradiation is a continuous process; therefore it is inevitable that products with different bulk densities will have to be adjacent to one another at some time or other on the conveyor. The conveyor speed to achieve a specified sterilizing dose differs between products of differing bulk densities. The greater the density, the slower the speed required to achieve a specific dose. Within the confines of some acceptable level of overdosing this situation is manageable. Every attempt must be made to minimize the density differences of products that must be run adjacent to one another, and any errors must be toward overdosing rather than underdosing.

Although the controlling factor in industrial irradiation is the conveyor speed, it is usual to supplement this by inclusion of dosimeters in the irradiator. The dosimeters are there as a confirmatory monitor that all factors remain under control. Routine dosimeters are not used as a control or a feedback system.

3. Dosimetry: Dose delivery in industrial-scale cobalt-60 gamma irradiators is achieved through controlling the time of exposure of the product to the source. The initial relationship between source strength, product bulk density, time of exposure, and absorbed dose has to be determined empirically by dosimetry.

Continued monitoring of dose as it might vary with adjustments to the time of exposure in response to source decay or product changes must also be done routinely using dosimeters.

Dosimetry is the measurement of absorbed dose. The unit of absorbed dose is the gray (Gy). Because dose is a measure of absorbed energy, calorimetry is the fundamental method of measurement. However, calorimetry suffers from being insensitive, complex, slow and highly demanding in technical skills and experience. Primary dose measurement is usually done with substances that are chemically changed quantitatively in response to the amount of radiation absorbed. For most purposes the standard primary system is the Fricke or ferrous sulfate dosimeter. In this system, which consists of a solution of ferrous sulfate in dilute sulfuric acid, ferrous ions Fe^{++} are oxidized by absorbtion of radiation to ferric ions Fe^{+++}. Fricke dosimeters are usually presented in glass ampoules; the yield of ferric ions is measured by UV spectrophotometry at 340 nm. They respond linearly to absorbed dose over the range 10 to 500 Gy, are accurate to about 1%, and show no dose rate dependence. Fricke dosimeters do not measure doses in the ranges seen in industrial-scale irradiators. They are, however, widely used for calibrating the radiation fields in national and international standards laboratories, which are in turn used to calibrate the types of dosimetry systems used in industrial-scale irradiators.

The types of dosimeter used most often for dose mapping and routine dose monitoring are referred to as secondary systems. This is because their response to radiation cannot be predicted from theoretical considerations. Instead, their response has to be calibrated from batch to batch and from time to time against a calibrated "standard" radiation field. The most commonly used types are made of dyed acrylic (mainly Harwell 4034 dosimeters). The overwhelming advantage of this type of dosimeter is its robustness. Table 5 highlights the differences between conditions in standards laboratories and those in industrial-scale irradiators. It is more important for dosimeters in routine use to give consistent results under variable conditions than to be highly accurate but environmentally sensitive and operator dependent. Harwell 4034 dyed acrylic dosimeters read out in the visible spectra at 640 nm; their range is 5 to 50 kGy, and their accuracy is around 5 to 10%.

It should be appreciated that there is a considerable difference between the dose ranges at which radiation fields are calibrated against Fricke dosimeters and the dose ranges for which the same fields are used to calibrate secondary dosimeters. These differences should be of no importance as long as neither of the dosimetry systems is dose rate dependent. However, it is not uncommon to find dosimeters that respond theoretically and quantitatively over wider ranges of dose being used in the commissioning of new irradiators and to supplement secondary dosimeter dose mapping after source replenishments. These are sometimes called transfer dosimeters because they may (theoretically but not usually practically) be used to calibrate radiation fields and also to monitor industrial-scale irradiators. Ceric-cerous (10 to 50 kGy) and potassium dichromate (1 to 100 kGy) dosimeters (both accurate to about 4%) are the most commonly used transfer dosimeters. Both, however, are liquid systems; readout can be potentiometric or by UV spectrophotometry, and a fair degree of skill is required in their use and handling. A solid-state system, alanine, which is accu-

Table 5 Comparison of Radiation Conditions Between Standard Sources and Industrial Irradiators

Factor	Standard source	Industrial irradiators
Dose rate	Constant	Variable
Temperature	Constant	Variable
Spatial distribution	Defined	Dependant upon product loading
Humidity	Constant	Variable
Storage of dosimeters before and after irradiation	Constant	May be variable

rate over the wider range of 1 Gy to 100 kGy, has been quoted as having a lot of promise [5]. The method of readout, electron spin resonance spectrophotometry, is neither straightforward nor cheap.

V. THE CHOICE OF DOSE

The question is, what is an appropriate sterilizing dose of radiation? Clearly, once a dose has been decided upon, the same general principles govern its delivery and its control irrespective of whether that dose is 10 kGy, 25 kGy or whatever. Are all products sterile if exposed to 25 kGy? Are there other more appropriate doses to achieve specified SALs? The answers to these questions are by no means simple. The underlying philosophies were reviewed in depth by Tallentire in 1983 [6]. As with most other sterilization technologies, the major schools of thought have split between process specifications and validated SALs. Since gamma irradiation is a fairly modern technology it is possible to trace the origins and the reasons behind the various options.

A. The 25 kGy "Standard" Dose

The first published reference to 25 kGy as an appropriate irradiation sterilization dose came from Artandi and Van Winkle in 1959 [7]. It did not come in the form of a general recommendation. It arose from technical considerations surrounding accelerated electron sterilization of catgut. These workers determined that catgut sutures could be irradiated to 50 kGy before showing properties inferior to those of heat-sterilized sutures. They also "established the minimum killing dose for over 150 species of microorganisms," and chose 25 kGy as their sterilizing dose because it was 40% above that necessary to kill the most resistant microorganism and well short of that which would damage the product. Just what they meant by a "minimum killing dose" was not explained within the technical content of the paper, but clearly the exponential nature of microbial inactivation was not taken into consideration.

By 1965, 25 kGy was quoted [8] as being the accepted dose of radiation for sterilizing disposable medical equipment in most countries except Denmark, where 45 kGy was being claimed to be necessary. As a consequence there was a flurry of scientific activity to validate the choice of 25 kGy retrospectively. Much of this work was done in laboratory studies with the most radiation-resistant microorganism then known, the spore of *Bacillus pumilus* E601 and centered on the determination of inactivation factors. An inactivation factor is the number of decimal reduction values (D_{10}-values) delivered by a particular dose. For these spores irradiated in air the D_{10} was consistently found to be 1.7 kGy, hence the inactivation factor was 15. This implies that an SAL of better than 10^{-6} can be achieved for items contaminated with up to 10^9 spores of these microorganisms per item, and by inference for higher bioburdens of less radiation-resistant microorganisms. However, under different environmental conditions microorganisms respond differently to radiation. Under anoxic (absence of oxygen) conditions of irradiation the D_{10} for spores of *Bacillus pumilus* E601 was consistently found to be 3.4 kGy, the inactivation factor for 25 kGy was therefore about 7, and the maximum bioburden per item that would support a 10^{-6} SAL was only about 10. Since anoxia is quite improbable in practical situations it was felt that these studies supported the view of 25 kGy as being a satisfactory "standard" sterilizing dose. Most regulatory agencies outside of the U.S.A. still prefer the "standard" 25 kGy standard dose with two provisos:

(a) It can only be used in conjunction with implementation of GMP (good manufacturing practices) in order to achieve a low bioburden prior to sterilization.

(b) Lower doses may may be acceptable if there is technical need, e.g., with dose-dependent deleterious effects on materials, and if there is evidence to validate the lower dose.

Somewhere around the confidence in a "standard" dose are the practicalities of it being simple and easy to administer by regulatory authorities, and of it being easy to justify by medical device manufacturers who may not be prepared to commit to the levels of microbiological effort required to validate other doses.

B. Irradiation in Scandinavia

In the 1960s the Danish authorities held that there should be a common standard of acceptance for all sterile products irrespective of method of sterilization. They were not initially basing this on a SAL of 10^{-6} but on an inactivation factor of 8, because this was their standard for thermal inactivation processes. Furthermore, they maintained that the microorganism to which the inactivation factor referred should be the most resistant type known, presented to the sterilization process under worst-case conditions. For irradiation, the reference microorganism was chosen to be a strain of *Streptococcus faecium* A2 with a shouldered inactivation curve irradiated in dried serum broth. The standard dose was set at 45 kGy.

The situation in Scandinavia eased in the 1970s. The *Nordic Pharmacopoeia* introduced the 10^{-6} SAL, and standard sterilizing doses were modified to take account of the average bioburden per item prior to sterilization. The minimum sterilizing dose was set at 32 kGy.

C. Irradiation in North America

Although all major pharmacopoeias now cite the 10^{-6} SAL for all methods of sterilization, the USP goes further in its recommendations concerning irradiation than its European counterpart. An approach to validation of the 10^{-6} SAL is indicated, via the Association for the Advancement of Medical Instrumentation's (AAMI) *Process Control Guidelines for Gamma Radiation Sterilization of Medical Devices, 1984* [9]. Several methods are described here but only two are being much used. These two methods share the same philosophy, that the most relevant approach to validation of a sterilization process is to consider the response to treatment (in this case irradiation) of the innate bioburden *in situ*. Arguments about the choice of reference microorganisms are thus avoided, as also are arguments about the relevance of laboratory "worst case" conditions to practical situations. The two methods are contained in Appendixes B1 and B2 to the *Process Control Guidelines*.

1. The AAMI B1 Method: The AAMI B1 method is based on inactivation of a hypothetical mixed culture of microorganisms. This hypothetical mixed culture contains microorganisms of various D_{10} values present in different defined frequencies; this is referred to as the "standard but arbitrary" distribution of radiation responses. Inactivation of populations of various different initial numbers, but always conforming to the "standard but arbitrary" distribution of radiation responses, was simulated by computer. From the simulation a series of tables was derived relating initial number of contaminants to dose and SAL.

Practically, the method first requires an estimate of average numbers of microorganisms on items. The contaminant population is assumed to respond to radiation in the same way as the "standard but arbitrary" distribution.

By reference to the tables in Appendix B1 of the *Guidelines*, doses of radiation appropriate to SALs of 10^{-2} and 10^{-6} can be determined. The second practical consideration is to test the hypothesis by irradiating one hundred items at the tabulated 10^{-2} dose. Unless the actual distribution of radiation sensitivities of the microorganisms on the items is more resistant than the "standard but arbitrary" distribution, then all one hundred items will be sterile when tested. This then supports the tabulated dose required to achieve a 10^{-6} SAL.

The method relies on four assumptions:

(a) The validity of the computer simulation. This is based on exponential inactivation, and on each component of a mixed culture responding independently of the others.

(b) The validity of the "standard but arbitrary" distribution of radiation responses. The data used to develop this distribution was taken from very limited studies. Nonetheless, the items from which the microorganisms were isolated were first given "screening" doses of radiation to eliminate very sensitive types. It is biased toward greater radiation resistance than one might be likely to encounter except in very unusual situations (for instance dried in serum broth).

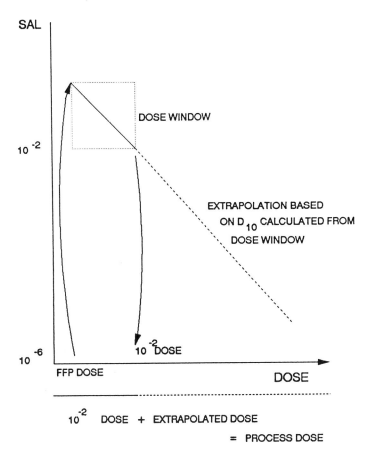

Fig. 4 Coordinates of the AAMI B2 dose setting method.

(c) The validity of the estimate of bioburden. This ought to be reliable, but in fact the method has a conservative bias because an overly low estimate of bioburden would give a commensurately low tabulated 10^{-2} dose and lead to failure in the irradiation trial.

(d) The validity of the method of testing the items for sterility after the irradiation trial. Adequate controls must be considered.

2. The AAMI B2 Method: The AAMI B2 method assumes far less than the AAMI B1 method. It assumes exponential inactivation. It does not assume any "standard but arbitrary" distribution and it does not require estimation of bioburden. It does, however, continue to require well controlled sterility testing methods, and it requires more elaborate experimental irradiation equipment than the B1 method.

The B2 method makes use of a series of nine doses of radiation that are only fractions of the probable process dose (sub-process doses) to determine two sets of coordinates of a functional relationship that describes inactivation of innate contaminants on product items. The first set of coordinates is for the dose that represents an average of three microorganisms per item. This (called the FFP or first fraction positive) is the lowest dose at which at least one item in a set of twenty is sterile. The second set of coordinates is for the dose at which a 10^{-2} SAL is achieved.

The region between the two sets of coordinates is called the "dose window" (Fig. 4). The response to radiation within the dose window is assumed to be exponential, and therefore a D_{10} can be calculated. The dose required to achieve an SAL of 10^{-6} is then derived from the 10^{-2} dose plus as many calculated D_{10} values as are required to achieve the target. The B2 method therefore recognizes that there may be two components to radiation sensitivities of a contaminant population: a sensitive portion that is addressed through determination of the actual 10^{-2} SAL dose and a more resistant "tail" population than is accounted for by extrapolation.

REFERENCES

1. Dunn, C. G., Campbell, W. L., Fram, H. and Hutchins, A. (1948). Biological and photochemical effects of high energy electrostatically produced roentgen rays and cathode rays. *Journal of Applied Physics* **19**: 605–616.
2. Tallentire, A. (1980). The spectrum of microbial radiation sensitivity. *Radiation Physics and Chemistry* **15**: 83–89.
3. Jacobs, G. P. (1985). A review: Radiation sterilization of pharmaceuticals. *Radiation Physics and Chemistry* **26**: 133.
4. Department of Health and Social Security (1981). *Guide to Good Manufacturing Practice for Medical Devices and Surgical Products, 1981.* London: Her Majesty's Stationery Office.
5. Miller, A., Chadwick, K. H. and Nam, J. W. (1983). Dose assurance in radiation processing plants. *Radiation Physics and Chemistry* **22**: 31–40.
6. Tallentire, A. (1983). Philosophies underlying sterility assurance of radiation-treated products. *Medical Devices and Diagnostics Industry* **5**: 36–42.
7. Artandi, C., and Van Winkle, W. (1959). Electron beam sterilization of surgical sutures. *Nucleonics* **17**: 86–90.
8. Ley, F. J., and Tallentire, A. (1965). Radiation sterilisation—The choice of *dose. Pharmaceutical Journal* **195**: 216–218.
9. Association for the Advancement of Medical Instrumentation (1984). *Process Control Guidelines for Gamma Radiation Sterilization of Medical Devices.* AAMI: Arlington, Virginia, U.S.A.

Sterilization by Saturated Steam

Sterilization by saturated steam under pressure is the classical time-proven and most economical method of inactivation of microorganisms. When a requirement for sterility arises for a new type of medical device or pharmaceutical product, steam should always be given first consideration. This is because, importantly, steam of the correct quality leaves no residues. Regrettably, it is unsuitable for heat-sensitive and moisture-sensitive products and packaging materials.

For the most part, steam raises the temperatures of objects that come into its contact by condensing on the cooler surfaces of the objects. In this way it loses latent heat to the object. This effect when applied to microorganisms results in death through coagulation of cellular proteins. This biochemical effect begins to be significant at moist heat temperatures above about 80°C and proceeds rapidly within the normal processing range of about 110°C to 140°C. This is quite different from the mechanism of inactivation of microorganisms by dry heat, which is mainly oxidative; as a consequence, the temperature ranges required by the two processes are quite distinct. Far higher temperatures are required from dry heat sterilization to achieve the same lethalities as those obtained with steam sterilization.

Microorganisms differ in their responses to high temperatures. The innate or inherent resistance to thermal inactivation of bacterial endospores is considerably higher than that of vegetative microorganisms. There are also considerable species-to-species differences within the spore-forming genera themselves. Much of the experimental work on thermal inactivation of microorganisms has therefore been done on the more heat-resistant spores because they have measureable variations in their responses to heat as well as being troublesome organisms with respect to their potential to survive heat processing. Although there are some distinct differences, the overall enzyme complements of heat-resistant spores and vegetative cells are broadly similar. This implies that there must be some factors within the spore to stabilize, protect, or repair essential heat-labile proteins that would not survive high temperatures if present in the vegetative cell. These factors are complex and subtle, but they clearly involve low water content, the presence of chelated metal ions, particularly Ca^{++}, the presence of dipicolinic acid, and enzymatic repair activity.

The first application of steam under pressure to microbial inactivation is usually attributed to Appert's food canning process. The principle of that method, namely the displacement of air by steam within a pressure vessel, usually termed an autoclave (or a retort in the canning industry), has remained substantially the same for over 100 years. The classical autoclave was set to operate at an internal pressure of 15 psig (approximately 1 atm above normal atmospheric pressure), affording a temperature of 121°C. There is nothing particularly significant about the pressure of 1 bar or the temperature of 121°C other than the availability of technology that can achieve these conditions and a conservative tendency to standardize thermal inactivation to conditions of known effectiveness. Modern autoclaves may be specified and constructed to operate over a range of internal pressures, providing different temperatures determined

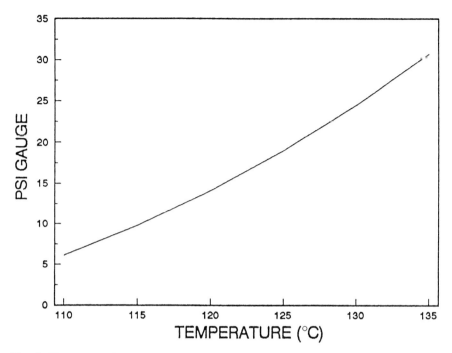

Fig. 1 Temperature/pressure equilibrium for steam.

by the temperature/pressure equilibria for steam (Fig. 1). Small-scale and large-scale technologies are available.

I. HEAT TRANSFER

The effectiveness of thermal inactivation rests with heat transfer from the steam to the microorganisms. Provided that there is a temperature difference between two parts of a system, heat flows from one part to the other by one, two or all three of three mechanisms:

(a) Conduction. In this mechanism heat is transferred from one substance to another by vibrational energy of atoms or molecules. There is no mixing of the two substances. Transfer of heat from an autoclave through the walls of a container or packaging material occurs by conduction. For liquids, further heat transfer by conduction is minimal.

(b) Convection. Convection only occurs in fluids. Heat transfer is by warm fluids mixing with cooler fluids. This mechanism is of significant importance to sterilization of fluid loads in autoclaves.

(c) Radiation. Radiant heat energy moves through space by means of electromagnetic waves. If radiant energy comes into contact with an object, heat is absorbed by the object or conducted through it. Radiant heat does not make a significant contribution to heat transfer in autoclaves, but it is important to dry heat sterilization (see Chapter 5).

Heat penetration into items being sterilized by saturated steam begins with the outside of each item (consider the items to be fluid containers) having a layer of condensed steam adhering to it. Transfer of heat is by conduction from the steam to the condensate, to the walls of the container, and on into the fluid. Each stationary boundary layer presents its own resistance to heat penetration. This resistance can be minimized by technologies that improve heat transfer, such as movement of the fluid within the containers or turbulence within the autoclave. Liquids have low thermal conductivities, but convection currents caused by local temperature gradients lead to continuous movements within the fluid, thus reducing the thermal resistance of the innermost boundary layer of the system. It is not usual to find sterilizer loads being agitated except in the case of rotary washer/autoclaves. It is quite usual on the other hand to find turbulence within the steam in the autoclave being achieved by fans or recirculation.

II. EFFECTS OF STEAM UNDER PRESSURE ON MICROBIAL POPULATIONS

Thermal damage to biological systems is caused by absorption of heat energy. Well-controlled laboratory studies show that when pure cultures of microorganisms are held in saturated steam at a constant sterilizing temperature there are linear relationships between the logarithm of the number of survivors and the time of exposure (exponential inactivation).

Figure 2 illustrates the terminology used for inactivation of microorganisms by saturated steam. The thermal resistances of particular microorganisms are expressed via the slopes of the exponential relationship. The D-value is the time in minutes (D_T) at a temperature T required to reduce the number of survivors by 90%. This relationship is described by an equation that is directly related to Eq. (2.3) in Chapter 2:

$$\log N_t = \frac{-t}{D} + \log N_0 \tag{4.1}$$

where N_0 = number of microorganisms prior to treatment, N_t = number of microorganisms surviving after time t expressed in minutes, and D = the D-value expressed in minutes.

It should be borne in mind that D_T-values relate specifically to the conditions under which they were determined. The immediate environment or sub-

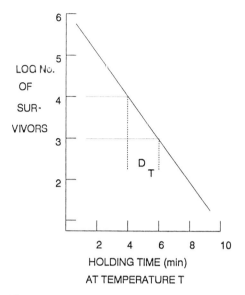

Fig. 2 *D*-values.

strate on which microorganisms are heated can have a significant effect on the microorganism's heat inactivation characteristics. There is a wealth of research data on this topic, for instance in connection with the physiological state of the microorganisms, in connection with pH, and in connection with the ionic composition of the environment. Some generalizations may be made, for instance thermal death rates are lowest at neutral pHs; proteinaceous materials and fats and oils are protective against heat inactivation. Nonetheless, in practical sterilization situations this type of information can only be supplementary to empirical data determined for particular products, packaging components, etc. Table 1 shows differences in *D*-values that can arise between spores of three different species of *Bacillus* on various substrates that might be associated with medical or pharmaceutical products.

The exponential relationship between numbers of surviving microorganisms and time of exposure at a particular temperature parallels first-order chemical kinetics. In these circumstances it should follow that equivalent lethalities at different temperatures of exposure should be predictable. When *D*-values have been determined for pure cultures of the same microorganism at different temperatures (Fig. 3), it has been shown that there is a linear relationship between the logarithm of the *D*-values and the temperatures at which they were determined $(T_1, T_2, T_3,$ etc.). The term *z* is given to the slope of this line; *z* is the number of degrees of temperature change necessary to alter the value of *D* by a

Table 1 Some D_{121}-Values Versus Saturated Steam of Bacterial Endospores Mounted in or on Various Substrates

	D_{121}-value (min)			
Spore	Distilled water	Glass	Rubber	Steel
B. stearothermophilus ATCC 7953	1.99	1.32	1.84	1.47
B. coagulans	0.99	—	0.80	—
B. subtilis	0.61	—	0.56	—

factor of 10. A z-value of 10°C is widely quoted for bacterial spores and is commonly used as a constant in computations of thermal lethality. An alternative to the z-value, most often quoted in academic texts, is the temperature coefficient or Q_{10}-value. This is defined as the change in rate of reaction brought about by a change in temperature of 10°C:

$$Q_{10} = \frac{D_{T+10}}{D_T} \tag{4.2}$$

where $D_T = D$-value determined at T°C and, $D_{T+10} = D$-value determined at T plus 10°C.

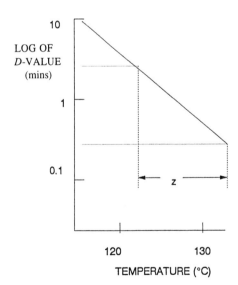

Fig. 3 z-Values.

Q_{10}-values in the range of 5 to 20 have been found for bacterial spores against saturated steam sterilizing temperatures. These rather high temperature coefficients show that for steam sterilization, a discrepancy of only 1 or 2°C from the specified temperature may have significant effects on the process lethality. For instance, a deficiency of 2 to 3°C could easily require a doubling of the exposure time to achieve the same lethality as the specified process.

A D-value accompanied by the temperature T at which it was determined and its z-value provide a complete definition of the heat inactivation characteristics D_T^z for any particular microorganism.

III. APPLICATIONS OF STEAM STERILIZATION

For an item to be suitable for steam sterilization it must be sufficiently heat-stable to withstand process temperatures. Further to this, it cannot be allowed to be susceptible to moisture damage, because sterilizing conditions will not be achieved in regions of the product that are not permeated by steam. Subject to these two constraints, products that are sterilizable by saturated steam fall into three categories, (a) aqueous liquids, (b) nonporous solids, and (c) porous solids.

A. Aqueous Liquids

There are several types of sterile aqueous pharmaceutical products—single-dose and multi-dose ophthalmics, and small-volume and large-volume multi-dose and single-dose parenterals. From necessity, all of these types of product are filled into hermetically sealed nonporous containers. Those products that are terminally sterilized by saturated steam may be contained within glass ampoules, glass vials, glass syringes, glass bottles, or flexible film infusion bags. There is no necessity for steam to penetrate into these containers nor come into contact with the product. As long as the sterilizing temperature is obtained, the water content of the product itself will be sufficient to ensure that microbial inactivation is due to moist heat protein coagulation mechanisms.

B. Nonporous Solids

Most solid dosage forms of parenteral pharmaceuticals are unsuitable for terminal steam sterilization. Many medical devices are nonporous solids, for instance scalpel blades and rubber catheters, and may, particularly in hospital-scale operations, be steam sterilized. Moist heat is usually the method of choice in laboratories and in industrial aseptic filling facilities for instruments and machine parts that are required to be sterile. This may apply even to equipment that is well able to withstand dry heat sterilization temperatures, for the sake of reducing the time involved in processing. In all cases it is critical that the items to be sterilized be hermetically sealed into containers that are capable of serving two functions, to allow steam to penetrate and come into contact with all parts of the product, and to provide effective barriers to microbial ingress while still intact. Papers made to specifications appropriate for steam sterilization are available for wrapping items and as made-up bags.

Rubber closures for vials or other containers being filled aseptically on an industrial scale are nonporous but share some of the problems of porous loads. They are most frequently steam sterilized by passage through double-ended rotary washer autoclaves, which by agitation of the product ensure effective steam penetration to even the potentially occluded parts of the closures. Steam comes into direct contact with these bulk items; they are not usually wrapped nor packed into hermetically sealed containers. Special precautions must be taken for unloading to avoid compromising their sterility. Static autoclaves may also be used for prewashed versions of these types of components. They should then be loaded into the autoclave in shallow layers in perforated trays or boxes.

C. Porous Solids

Sterile dressings, filters, and cellulosic materials in general are porous materials. It is generally problematic to ensure steam contact with all parts of porous materials because of entrapped air. Sterilizing temperatures will not be achieved in the presence of air. The mechanism of microbial inactivation in the presence of air will be that of dry heat, which is much slower than that of saturated steam. Avoidance of entrapped air is addressed through specific porous-load sterilization cycles rather than through any special packing or loading provision other than those constraining the sterilization of other solid products.

IV. AUTOCLAVES AND AUTOCLAVE CYCLES

The simplest autoclave is the domestic pressure cooker. Steam is generated within the pressure cooker. Air is allowed to discharge through the vent until "pure" steam only is seen to be emerging. The vent is sealed by a weighted valve. Pressure and temperature increase within the pressure cooker until the weighted valve begins to lift. The heat is turned down and the whole setup is left to simmer at the temperature dictated by the pressure within the cooker. All laboratory and production autoclaves, and washer/autoclaves, branch from this stem. There are five specific cycle stages seen for the domestic pressure cooker that must be addressed in the technology of all autoclaves: (a) air removal, (b) heat-up, (c) hold time, (d) drying, and (e) cooling.

A. Downward-Displacement Autoclaves

Many autoclaves will be of the downward-displacement (gravity-displacement) type. They operate on the principle of air being more dense than steam. As steam is admitted to the sterilizer, air is displaced downward and out of the sterilizer via a drain at the bottom.

Figure 4 represents a longitudinal section through a downward displacement autoclave and its associated pipework. It consists of an inner steel chamber surrounded by a steam jacket. Jackets are optional. Good insulation is an alternative. The objective of jacketing and/or other forms of insulation is to speed up the cycle by minimizing the need to heat up the mass of metal of the vessel itself, to prevent condensation forming on the vessel's internal walls, and to help speed up drying of the load at the end of the cycle.

Steam is supplied at high pressure from a steam generator to the jacket and directly to the rear of the chamber via a reducing valve. The incoming steam hits a baffle placed to prevent wetting of the load. Because it is hotter and lighter than air, the steam moves immediately upward and stratifies above the air in the chamber. With increasing pressure the steam forces the air out through the drain at the bottom of the chamber. A temperature sensor is strategically located at the coolest point in the drain line. The exposure period should be timed from when the equilibrium temperature that is correct for the pressure at which the autoclave has been set to operate is achieved in the drain line. It is quite usual to find modern autoclaves equipped with "floating" temperature sensors that can be located in the chamber or in the load itself. Nonetheless it is the drain sensor that is normally slowest to reach the set sterilizing temperature and is therefore critical for control purposes.

Modulation of the supply of steam to the chamber during heat-up and exposure may be achieved by thermostatic feedback from the drain line or through pressure transducers in the chamber.

B. High-Vacuum Autoclaves

The main factor accounting for lack of reliable attainment of sterility in autoclaves has been entrapped air acting as a barrier to direct contact between steam and product. Thus the main thrust for technological advances in steam sterilization has been concerned with improved effectiveness of removal of air from the chamber and its contents. Advanced high vacuum autoclaves have evolved from downward-displacement types by the addition of condensors, vacuum pumps, and ejector systems to assist in air removal.

The first stage in a high-vacuum cycle is to evacuate the loaded chamber. Some cycles may require a single evacuation, others may require a pulsing cycle of evacuation followed by steam injection repeated several times. The nature of the load dictates the cycle. Evacuation may be controlled through a pressure switch or transducer or simply by a timer governing pump running time. It is usual to find a condensor positioned between the chamber and the pump for purposes of pump protection.

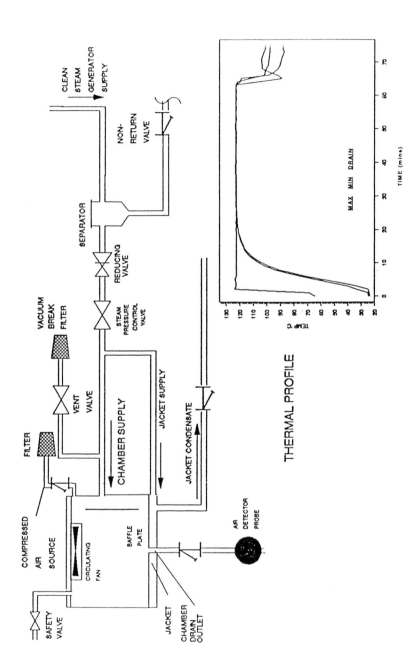

Fig. 4 Downward displacement autoclave and associated pipework.

High vacuum autoclaves are also usually equipped with air detector probes located in the pipework adjacent to the autoclave and linked to the cycle control instrumentation. During the cycle the temperature of the steam/air mixture is constantly monitored against a preset lower tolerance indicating unacceptable levels of air.

A typical high vacuum cycle for a nonporous solid load is illustrated in Fig. 5.

1. Porous Loads—Pulsed Cycles: Of all types of autoclave load, porous materials present the most serious problems of air removal. Air acts as an insulator and therefore impedes the condensation of steam on microorganisms and reduces process lethality. A further problem is that it is necessary that porous dressing packs and other cellulosic materials be completely dry at cycle completion.

These problems are usually addressed through pulsed cycles. Figure 6 shows a typical porous load pulsed cycle in which air removal takes place over five pulsed evacuations, each evacuating the chamber to a negative pressure of minus one bar (gauge). The first evacuation removes a large percentage of the air from the chamber. Evacuation is followed by injection of steam to atmospheric pressure; the steam mixes with the remaining air and to some extent preheats the load. Most of the remaining air is removed from the load by four repetitions of this vacuum pulse. Following the vacuum pulses, the cycle is set for four pulsed injections of steam to a preset positive pressure. The first purpose of these "positive" pulses is preheating, but they also contribute to mopping

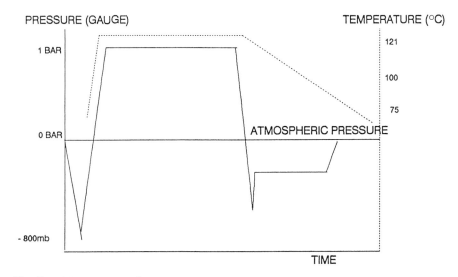

Fig. 5 High-vacuum cycle.

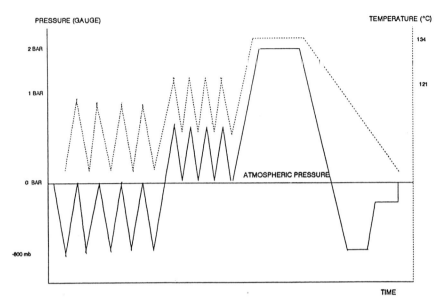

Fig. 6 Porous load pulsed cycle.

up any air remaining in the chamber or in the load. Cycle exposure is timed from when a "floating" load temperature sensor and the air detector probe reach the specified set temperature. The importance of the air detector probe in porous load cycles cannot be overemphasised.

At the end of the exposure period the chamber is evacuated to facilitate drying. During the drying phase, heat from the jacket helps to "flash" off condensate as the pressure drops.

2. Fluid Loads—Ballasted Cycles: Heat penetration into volumes of fluid tends to be slow. This is because aqueous products in primary containers usually have a very small surface area relative to their volume. Heat must be conducted through the walls of containers that are most often made from materials like glass or plastic, which are intrinsically poor conductors of heat. Thereafter, uniform temperatures in the fluid are dependent upon convection of heat within the containers.

The consequence of slow heat penetration is that the greater part of fluid load autoclave cycles is spent in bringing the load up to the exposure temperature and cooling it down again. For a particular autoclave, product, product container, and load configuration there is not much that can be done about the heat-up time. If the product is at all heat sensitive it is often practical to take account of the contribution made toward microbial lethality during heat-up as well as at the exposure temperature rather than risking product deterioration from overlong exposure. In some instances, particularly for large-volume parenteral products, the total cycle time can be reduced by accelerated chilled water cooling of the product after exposure. Alternatively, some autoclaves may be equipped with heat exchangers and forced draft fans within the chamber to assist rapid cooling.

Some types of container for liquid products, for instance glass ampoules, are sufficiently robust to withstand the rigors of steam sterilization under pressure. Sterilization cycles for ampoules are generally uncomplicated. However, other types of container are not as robust as ampoules and require rather more elaborate sterilization considerations. With stoppered vials, screw-cap bottles, flexible bags, and filled syringes there may be a significant increase in internal pressure within the headspace above the fluid during autoclaving. These internal pressures may result in closures and plungers being blown out. When a closure is completely blown out a product item becomes obviously unusable; perhaps more dangerously, a partially displaced closure may compromise the sterile barrier and go unnoticed. These difficulties may be avoided by use of air-ballasted (air overpressure) sterilization cycles.

In ballasted cycles the increase in pressure within the headspace of the container is counterbalanced with an internal chamber air overpressure. Figure 7 illustrates an idealized type of ballasted cycle; the autoclave operates as for a normal fluid load cycle up to the point at which the exposure temperature is attained (in this case 121°C or one bar [gauge] steam pressure), and then com-

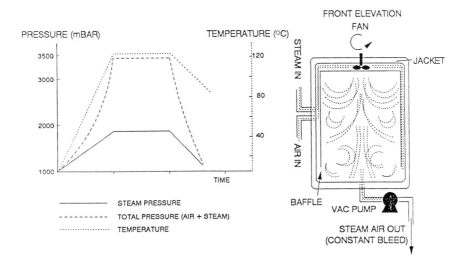

Fig. 7 Ballasted autoclave and cycle.

pressed air is injected into the chamber to a final pressure of 2.6 bar (gauge). At the end of the exposure period the pressure of 2.6 bar is maintained with compressed air only until cooling is complete. Ballasting pressure is usually maintained with air until all temperature probes register no more than 90°C; this is to ensure that closures will not be displaced in some parts of the load as a result of uneven cooling.

In practice, ballasting must take place before the exposure temperature is reached. It happens throughout the heating phase to compensate for the increases in internal pressure that accompany the increases in temperature. Different technologies address this differently in terms of the number of increments occurring during heat-up. There may be only as few as two or three steps, in each of which air is injected first, followed by steam to predetermined intermediate temperature and pressure equilibria. On the other hand, the modulation of internal pressure with increasing temperature may be virtually continuous in many tiny increments.

The pressure required to counterbalance internal headspace pressures may be determined empirically (Figure 8) or calculated from theoretical modelling. If done empirically, some care should be taken in relation to the amount of dead space in the system connecting the vessel under study to the pressure gauge, if erroneous results are to be avoided. This is particularly important for small headspaces and large dead spaces.

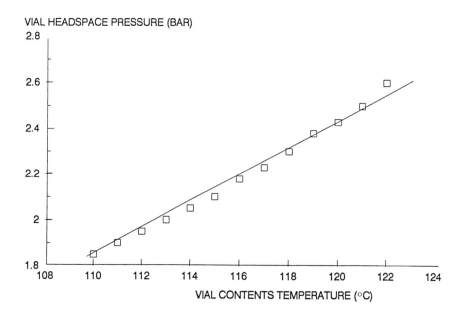

Fig. 8 Measurement of vial headspace pressure.

A theoretical model was described by Allwood [1] that proposes an equation for determining the internal pressure within a container in psia:

$$P_{T2} = \frac{P_0 V_1 T_2}{V_2 T_1} + \text{Vapor pressure within the container} \qquad (4.3)$$

where P_{T2} = internal pressure at exposure temperature T_2 ($^\circ K$); P_0 = assumed standard atmospheric pressure, 14.7 psia; T_1 = assumed temperature of liquid at time of filling, 20°C or 293°K; V_1 = (Headspace volume at T_1 + Volume of H_2O in headspace at T_1 – water vapor in air at T_1); and V_2 = Headspace volume at T_1 – Volume of expansion of liquid at T_2.

The important constraints within this model are the headspace volume above the liquid in the container and the volume of liquid in the container itself. Typically, larger ratios between headspace volumes and fluid volumes lead to higher internal pressures.

Joyce and Lorenz [2] presented a theoretical model based on similar principles. Table 2 summarizes the theoretical conclusions from this model over a temperature range of 116 to 121°C against fill volumes of 1 to 90%.

Both theoretical models and the empirical data shown in Fig. 8 reach broadly similar conclusions with regard to the pressure developing within closed containers raised to steam sterilization temperatures.

Table 2 Calculated Internal Pressures (psia) for Joyce and Lorenz [2]

Fill (%)	Temperature (°C)					
	116	117	118	119	120	121
	Pressure (psia)					
1	44.4	45.2	46.2	47.1	48.1	49.0
25	44.6	45.5	46.4	47.3	48.3	49.3
50	45.3	46.2	47.1	48.1	49.1	50.1
75	47.7	48.7	49.7	50.7	51.7	52.8
90	60.9	62.3	63.8	65.3	66.8	68.3

3. *Rotary Drum Washer/Autoclaves*: It is normal practice in large-scale aseptic filling of pharmaceutical products for vial closures to be sterilized into the aseptic filling room via double-ended washer/autoclaves. Figure 9 is a representation of a rotary drum washer/autoclave and its processing cycle. The setup has some resemblance to a domestic automatic washing machine except that the drum rotates rather more slowly. The whole chamber fills with water during the washing phase, the water is pumped out after the final rinse, and autoclaving proceeds as normal.

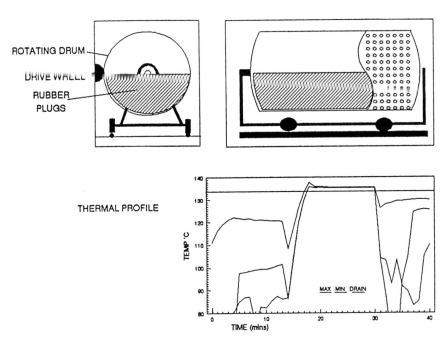

ROTATING DRUM

DRIVE WHEEL

RUBBER
PLUGS

THERMAL PROFILE

Fig. 9   Rotary drum washer/autoclave.

It is not possible within these autoclaves to operate with temperature probes within the load because of damage to the probes caused by the rotation. Since vial closures are sterilized in bulk and because it is undesirable to hold them in aseptic areas for lengthy periods of time before use, the possibility of using biological indicators as routine controls is also unacceptable. This places great emphasis on proper validation of these cycles and indeed on the design of vial closures. Vial closures of some designs can all too easily nest within one another, thus creating surfaces to which steam cannot penetrate. Autoclaves of this type should be equipped with mechanisms that ensure that they cannot operate unless the drum is rotating, or at the very least alarm signals should be displayed on the autoclave and on the permanent record in the event of drum failure.

4. Double-Ended Autoclaves: In many industrial applications autoclaves will be "bridges" between areas with different cleanliness classifications. The two main scenarios are that of an autoclave being loaded in a nonsterile preparation area for its sterilized contents to be unloaded in an aseptic filling room; and of an autoclave being loaded in a clean filling room for its sterilized contents to be unloaded into an uncontrolled packing area. In either example the risk is compromising the status of the clean side if both doors are open at the same time. Clearly, these double-ended autoclaves must be equipped with special interlocks and precautionary devices to prevent this from happening.

The two doors of double ended autoclaves should be interlocked in such a way that it is impossible to have both open at the same time. If there is no need to bridge areas, it is cheaper and simpler to purchase single-ended autoclaves. If possible, double-ended autoclaves should be unidirectional. It should only be possible to open the doors at one end of the autoclave by operating controls at that end. This means that a loading operator should not be able to open the unloading doors by some remote means, and the same applies to the unloader. In other words, the equipment should dictate that the staff in each area be wholly responsible for their own access to the autoclave in their respective areas.

There should be automatic signals at both ends of the autoclave indicating *doors locked* when both doors are locked and secure. Other signals at both ends should include a device indicating *sterilizing* during the whole cycle and *cycle complete* when the cycle is over. This is to allow staff on both sides to know the status of the autoclave and prevent any misguided attempts at entry. Once the loading door has been closed, it should not be possible to open the unloading door until the autoclave has satisfactorily completed a sterilization cycle. This is to prevent an autoclave being loaded with nonsterile items and then being unloaded without them having gone through any form of processing.

5. Autoclave Control Systems: Modern production-scale autoclaves are usually computer controlled. Older models may be electromechanically controlled (hardwired). Manual control is rare, and much of the knowledge and many of the skills required in the past to operate autoclaves successfully are being lost to turnkey operation. In many respects this is a giant leap forward to more consistent assurance of sterility. A genuine concern is that some will think that computer-controlled autoclaves are foolproof; indeed, they are not.

It is important to know how particular autoclaves work and to know how particular cycles are controlled. The software in computer-controlled autoclaves should be inviolable; it should have been validated, and it should respond in a predictable manner to signals received, sending out only the correct response signals and verifying that what was meant to happen actually did happen. However, somewhere in the loop there will be sensors, switches, valves, and pieces of miscellaneous plumbing. Murphy's law, which states that anything that can go wrong will go wrong, applies to these systems, and unless they are well understood by sterilization scientists as well as by engineers, electricians, and mechanics, the risk is nonsterility.

Autoclave control systems respond to three types of signal, time, temperature, and pressure. By far the most reliable of these is time, because of the intrinsic reliability of quartz timing devices. Temperature sensors are quite reliable but respond more slowly than pressure transducers. Pressure may be controlled by pressure switches that are activated (or deactivated) at one specific pressure only, or by pressure transducers that respond and send signals over calibrated ranges of pressures. Pressure sensors are electromechanical devices depending upon movement of flexible diaphragms to convert pressure signals into electrical pulses.

Usually only one phase of a sterilization cycle is controlled by time, and that is the exposure or temperature hold phase. Once the sterilizing temperature is reached and registered by the computer, the purpose of the timer is to signal stop to any further steam injections after the appropriate elapsed time. In essence this timed phase has a one-tailed error. If the signal is sent, the worst from the standpoint of sterility that can happen is that it is ignored and the sterilization phase will be protracted. This is not a problem from the sterilization standpoint unless the effect of heat damages the hermetic enclosure of the items being sterilized.

Time signals, because of their reliability, may be used to support other phases of autoclave cycles. So-called "phase time excesses" may be built into preliminary vacuum phases, heat-up phases, and cooling phases. A phase time excess is an alarm condition raised in response to a particular phase of the sterilization cycle happening faster or (more typically) slower than expected. Phase time excess alarms may provide essential indications of vacuum pump failure or sticking air or steam valves. The more complex the cycle, the greater the need to confirm that the validated condition is being replicated in routine use.

Temperature signals are used for several purposes. First, they are always used to signal that the sterilizing temperature has been reached. Two or more sensors should be used for this purpose, and the timed exposure phase should not be started until all of the sensors reach specification.

In some autoclaves, temperature signals are used to modulate the temperature within its specified band during the exposure period. In such cases the signal via the computer is directed to a steam valve that opens in response to a low temperature signal and closes in response to a high-temperature signal.

It is quite usual to find a high internal pressure maintained in autoclaves at the end of their sterilization phases until some cooling has taken place. This is typical for fluid load cycles, which may be held under air pressure until the signals from all of the sensors indicate that the temperature is lower than 80°C. In these cases the signal is to close the air injection valve and open a pressure release valve at the appropriate temperature. Cooling may be subject to a phase time excess.

Many phases of an autoclave cycle may be controlled through pressure signals. Pumping down to preliminary vacuums continues until pressure signals isolate the pump and open a steam valve. The sterilization hold phase may also be controlled by pressure signals. The pressure at which the specified temperature was reached may be maintained within limits of pressure (and hence of temperature) by pressure signals to the steam valve. With current technology, pressure signals afford finer control of temperature within the sterilization phase of autoclave cycles than temperature signals.

C. Steam Quality and Superheating

Since microbial lethality is a function of the latent heat of steam being discharged during condensation, it follows that the steam itself should be of a suitable quality to ensure that maximum energy is available. Ideally, this is "dry" saturated steam supplied from a steam generator located close to the point of use. A less than ideal situation is for the boiler house to be a long way from the autoclave, thereby allowing the steam to condense and pick up excessive amounts of water droplets before reaching the autoclave. This makes it necessary to incorporate moisture traps in the steam lines and ensure that all pipework is well insulated or traced if wet loads resulting from the condensation of water in the steam are to be avoided.

A second area of concern associated with steam quality is superheating. This is a phenomenon related to the phase equilibria of steam under pressure (Fig. 1). In some circumstances it is possible at a fixed pressure to increase the temperature of steam above its equilibrium temperature. It is then referred to as superheated or supersaturated steam. Superheated steam is not as effectively lethal to microorganisms as saturated steam—the biochemical mechanisms of lethality are similar to those of dry heat. If supersaturated conditions prevail, the lethality of the process will be much lower at any specified temperature than that which would be expected from saturated steam. Supersaturation may arise from autoclave problems or load problems or both. For instance, the steam in the chamber may pick up heat from a jacket running at too high a temperature or pressure, or condensation of the steam may be impeded by very dry cellulosic materials in the load.

V. TEMPERATURE/TIME CRITERIA FOR STERILIZATION

Microbial lethality from steam sterilization is a function of two parameters, temperature and time. The choice of a cycle is ultimately dependent upon the heat-stability of the product, the type of primary container, the knowledge of heat penetration into the product, the autoclave technology available, and the knowledge of the microbiological contamination prior to sterilization. However, the pharmacopoeias (particularly the USP) offer some sound general advice to the selection of criteria.

The classic pharmacopoeial approach to steam sterilization has been the compendial cycle. Compendial cycles are described in terms of process specifications, for instance 15 min at 121°C (USP/EP/BP) and 134°C for 3 min (BP compendial cycle for dressings). The specified temperatures and times are for the exposure period and make no allowance for lethality contributed by heat-up and cool-down phases of the sterilization cycle. Historically, a claim to sterility could be made for a batch of items that could be shown to have undergone a compendial cycle, and from which an inappropriately small number of items had been shown to pass a pharmacopoeial sterility test. This is no longer the case, and although compendial cycles remain a viable option for steam sterilization cycles, most responsible sterilizers and all regulatory agencies will require further supportive evidence that even the compendial cycles are really capable of assuring sterility.

Beyond the compendial cycle, the next level of sophistication is the overkill cycle. Overkill cycles are based on inactivation factors and therefore share a common origin with the "botulinum cook" of the canning industry. The USP states, "a lethality input of $12D$ may be used in a typical overkill approach." Clearly some knowledge of D-values is necessary to apply this approach; for reference and in the absence of further information a D_{121} for spores of *Bacillus stearothermophilus* may be used. The USP quotes a D_{121} of 1.5 min. Using this information, an overkill cycle would be set as 18 min exposure at 121°C. With local detailed knowledge, a D-value for the most heat-resistant microorganisms actually contaminating a particular product may be substituted for that of *B. stearothermophilus* in establishing an appropriately longer or shorter overkill cycle.

Overkill cycles, however, take no account of the numbers of microorganisms contaminating product items. Consequently, an overkill cycle for a heavily contaminated product will not differ from that for a similar but far more lightly contaminated product. In 1980 the USP first formally recognized the now-standard sterility assurance level (SAL) of 10^{-6} (i.e., assurance of less than one chance in 1,000,000 that a sterilized item is microbiologically contaminated) as a legitimate target for sterilization processes. However, application of the SAL approach to determining sterilization cycles requires much more microbiological information than the compendial cycle approach or the overkill approach, namely an actual knowledge of the numbers of microorganisms contaminating product items. This practical information may then be coupled with a D-value (assumed for a reference microorganism or determined for actual heat-resistant contaminants) and used to determine an appropriate cycle. For instance, product items contaminated at an average level of 100 colony-forming units per item, with all contaminants assumed to have a D_{121}-value of 0.75 min, would be assured of an SAL of 10^{-6} by an exposure of 6 min at 121°C.

The move away from compendial cycles to overkill and SAL cycles went hand in hand with an increasing interest in the concept of equivalent lethalities being obtainable from different temperature/time combinations—the F_0 concept.

The F_0 concept originated from laboratory studies of the type summarized in Fig. 2 and Fig. 3, which show that a particular lethal effect can be obtained through different combinations of time and temperature. The F_0 value is a reference point to lethality at 121°C. F_0 values are expressed in minutes. An F_0 value of however many minutes tells you that the particular combination of temperature and time being used has equivalent lethality to that number of minutes at 121°C. The F_0 concept allows valid cycles based on times at 121°C to be translated into other temperature and time combinations equally valid.

At one time, the pharmacopoeias were specifying a standard F_0 value of 8 min for steam sterilization regardless of load type, presterilization microbiological contamination levels, or product stability. The last editions of the major pharmacopoeias in which an F_0 of 8 appeared were the 1980 USP and the 1988 BP. An F_0 of 8 means that the sterilizing cycle being used has an equivalent lethality to 8 min at 121°C.

The focus of recent editions of the pharmacopoeias is that an F_0 should be sufficient to assure an SAL of 10^{-6}. The F_0 value may be calculated for the timed exposure period only, but it is more commonly computed from the total accumulated lethal heat input above 80°C.

The following equation may be used to calculate simple F_0 values:

$$F_0 = D_{121} (\log A - \log B) \qquad (4.4)$$

where F_0 = minimum lethality, assuming z to equal 10°C; A = number of viable microorganisms per item prior to sterilization; and B = SAL.

Equivalent times at other temperatures may be calculated from the following equation [3]:

$$F_T^z = \frac{F_{121}^z}{L} \qquad (4.5)$$

where F_T^z = the equivalent time at temperature T to achieve a specified lethality for contaminants with a specified z-value, F_{121}^z = the equivalent time at 121°C to achieve the same specified lethality (when z is equal to 10°C, $F_{121}^z = F_0$),

$$L = \text{lethal rate } (10[T - 121]/z) \qquad (4.6)$$

F_0 values for the accumulated heat input during heat-up, exposure, and cool-down portions of a sterilization cycle may be obtained by plotting the lethal rates obtained at successive time intervals during the sterilization cycle against time, and determining the area under the curve.

Mathematically this is expressed as

$$F_0 = L \, dt \qquad (4.7)$$

Various methods are available for performing this integration (see Pflug [4]), but nowadays F_0 values are invariably integrated automatically with standard sterilizer monitoring equipment (for instance the Kaye Digistrip). Such equipment usually assumes D_{121} to be equal to 1 min, and z to be equal to 10°C.

VI. VALIDATION AND CONTROL OF STEAM STERILIZATION

A. Validation

Validation of a steam sterilization process must cover the series of actions required to establish that the process is capable of doing what it is intended to do (i.e., supporting a claim of sterility) and must define a plan for maintaining the validated state of control. An overall scheme is described in Table 3.

In an ideal world, sterilization validation begins even before the purchase of an autoclave. Although this would appear to belong mainly with the engineering side of sterilization, it is also of major importance to the operational and control side too. A sterilization cycle must be tailored to each product and its container/closure system, so it is best to have first defined the range of potential applications, to be sure that new equipment is correctly specified. On installation, the autoclave should be checked out to ensure that it meets its specification, that it has been properly installed, and that its instrumentation is within calibration.

Thereafter, the new autoclave must be validated and scheduled for routine revalidation, maintenance, and recalibration at appropriate intervals. Since the

Table 3 Essentials of Steam Sterilization Validation

SPECIFICATION	*Must define* chamber size, construction quality, control systems, operating parameters, cycle operations, requirement for services, safety systems, machine/building interface.
INSTALLATION	*Must ensure that the autoclave* is located in a bounded area to control water leaks, has good access for maintenance, has an air-break in the drain line, has sample ports for steam and water testing, is located in an area that allows for heat dissipation.
COMMISSIONING	*Must demonstrate* that all operating systems are working, that all safety systems are working, that the autoclave has been tested for leaks and other malfunctions, that there is cycle to cycle continuity of performance. *Must include* calibration of all control equipment.
VALIDATION	*Must demonstrate* good heat distribution in empty chambers for all proposed cycles and good heat penetration studies for all proposed loads. *Must determine* ongoing operating specification. *Must establish* a calibration program for all equipment involved in controlling or monitoring performance, a program for routine maintenance.

critical parameters of sterilization by saturated steam are known, and the effects of saturated steam on microorganisms in general are well documented, the main thrust for autoclave validation is to ensure that the specified temperature is achieved in all parts of the autoclave and throughout the load. Biological validation is secondary to thermal validation except in circumstances where it is considered that thermal data is unreliable.

Thermal profiles should demonstrate uniformity of temperature throughout empty chambers and from cycle to cycle. Any cold spots should be identified and if possible corrected at this stage of validation. Since revalidation must become a regular occurrence, new sterilizers should be specified with access glands for the thermocouples used for this purpose. Data from the thermocouples should be logged by a suitable multichannel recorder such as the Kaye Digistrip, which also computes cumulative F_0 values when temperatures exceed 80°C. Significant advances are being made in the field of computerized data logging systems, particularly with regard to information presentation and data storage.

Particular load configurations must be specified in detail and documented. The loading pattern of an autoclave can have significant effects on heat distribution and penetration. The second phase of thermal validation is to demonstrate uniformity of heat penetration throughout specimen loads (thermal load profiles). For this purpose temperature sensors must be located within the items being sterilized. All loading patterns should be evaluated, and good replication should be evident from cycle to cycle for the same pattern. Once again cold spots (if any) should be identified and loading patterns modified to minimize them. Specified F_0 values for particular products must be achieved in the coldest part of the load.

In the case of porous loads it may be valuable to perform heat distribution studies on fully loaded autoclaves to provide additional assurance with regard to air removal and thermal uniformity.

These thermal studies are the basis of validation and ongoing revalidation of autoclaves.

In some instances they may need to be supplemented by microbiological validation, but this should be seen as the exception rather than the rule. There may be reason to believe that thermal data from load profile studies are overoptimistic; perhaps steam may be penetrating into the load along channels created by the thermocouple wires. Moreover, there may be reason to believe that dry heat conditions are prevailing in some parts of the load; for instance, it is not unknown for some types of vial closure plugs to nest one inside another in rotary washer/autoclaves. Steam cannot penetrate to the occluded surfaces, and nonsterile plugs may be discharged. In these cases biological studies are the only means of ascertaining whether true sterilizing conditions exist.

Spores of *B. stearothermophilus* ATCC 7953 (or CIP 52.81 or NCTC 10007 or NCIB 81 57) or *Clostridium sporogenes* ATCC 7955 (or NCTC 8594 or NCIB 8053) are the recognized biological test pieces for sterilization by saturated steam. They may be purchased as spore suspensions that can be inoculated onto test pieces of one's own choosing, or as ready-made test pieces on paper or aluminum strips. An incubation temperature of 55°C should be used to test for viability after exposure.

B. Routine Control

Academic texts on steam sterilization often state that routine control of steam sterilization processes should concentrate on the measurable determinants of lethality, temperature and time. Temperature should be monitored at the coldest point, usually in the drain line, but if this is not the coldest spot there should be a "floating" probe at the coldest spot, or the relationship between the drain line and the coldest spot should have been well established and documented. A permanent record of the temperature throughout the sterilization cycle should be a compulsory feature of all production-scale autoclaves, and this should be inspected in detail for batch release. In practice this is not sufficient to confirm that sterilizing conditions have been attained.

Sterilization by saturated steam is only effective for particular combinations of temperature and time in the absence of air. Permanent records of pressure should also be inspected as part of routine batch release. Deviations from the known equilibrium that exists for steam between temperature and pressure may be indicators of superheating. Inspection of the pressure traces of the preliminary phases of sterilization cycles may reveal faulty steam or vacuum valves, which could impact upon sterility assurance. Presterilization temperature traces are often too messy to be meaningful in these phases of sterilization cycles. This is due to differences between hot and cold starts, differences in temperature between probes in one part of the load and another, etc.

Where modern autoclaves can provide analog and digital records of temperature and pressure against time, both should be provided in the permanent record and inspected diligently before product release. Manual transcription of process conditions from dial or digital gauges is not an acceptable approach to control of autoclaves.

Routine biological monitors are still being used as routine controls in the U.S.A., but very rarely in Europe. With modern technology these should not be necessary.

For porous loads, two other monitoring techniques are in use to give assurance of sterility where there is a risk of air entrainment, superheating, etc. These are the Bowie-Dick test pack and the Lantor Cube. It should be emphasized that these are used in rather special applications and would be of little significance to fluid loads or nonporous solid loads.

1. The Bowie-Dick Test Pack: The Bowie-Dick standard test pack consists of a series of folded stacked towels. Strips of heat-sensitive tape are placed from corner to corner to form a Saint Andrew's cross pattern at various depths within the pack. The towels are fairly tightly wrapped, sealed with tape and placed in the autoclave along with a routine load.

The indicator tape changes color from light to dark when moist heat sterilizing conditions prevail. In the presence of air the tape does not darken. Well-outlined unchanged areas can be seen on the tape in areas where air has been entrained.

2. The Lantor Cube: The Lantor cube was developed as a reusable and more reliable alternative to the Bowie-Dick towel pack. It consists of a 15 cm cube of laminated polypropylene supplied in two halves. A sheet of paper carrying strips of heat-sensitive indicator tape is placed between the two sections of the cube and clamped in place. Interpretation is the same as for the Bowie-Dick test pack.

C. Some Autoclave Problems

The autoclave, like any other piece of industrial equipment, suffers problems that are not wholly addressed by preventative maintenance programs. Some of these may affect production, some may affect sterility, some may have an effect on both. Some of the difficulties that most autoclave operators periodically encounter are listed in the next few sentences. The consequence of most of these can be avoided by regular inspection and constant vigilance.

Sometimes drain outlets get blocked with broken glass or other such debris, thereby preventing free removal of air and accumulation of condensate in the chamber.

Door seals perish. The consequence is that pressure cannot be maintained and sterilizing temperatures are not reached. If not diagnosed through other symptoms, perished door seals should be detected in periodic leak rate performance checks. These checks should be performed with a greater regularity than thermal validation but are arguably not part of routine control of the autoclave. The leak check is an indicator of the airtightness of the chamber and associated pipework during a cycle. The test involves pulling a deep vacuum; the pump is then turned off and the vacuum held for a set time, usually 15 min. The pressure increase in the vessel should not exceed a specified small amount over the whole of the hold period.

Temperature probes are damaged. Records become unavailable. Feedback is interrupted.

Wet loads arise from poor steam quality or progressive pump deterioration, resulting in slow evacuation or inadequate vacuums during cooling.

Operator error results in products being loaded in the wrong configuration, or the wrong cycle is selected for a particular product load.

REFERENCES

1. Allwood, M. C., Hambleton, R., and Beverley, S. (1975). Pressure changes in bottles during sterilization by autoclaving. *Journal of Pharmaceutical Sciences* **64** (2): 333–334.
2. Joyce, M. A. and Lorenz, J. W. (1990). Internal pressure of sealed containers during autoclaving. *Journal of Parenteral Science and Technology* **44**: 320–323.
3. Parenteral Drug Association (1978). *Technical Monograph No. 1. Validation of Steam Sterilization Cycles.* Parenteral Drug Association: Washington, D.C., U.S.A.
4. Pflug, I. J. (1973). Heat sterilization. In *Industrial Sterilization* (G. Briggs Phillips and W. S. Miller, eds.). Duke University Press: Durham, N.C., U.S.A.

ANNEX 1. CALCULATING CONTAINER INTERNAL PRESSURES FOR A FILLED SYRINGE TO BE STERILIZED IN A 115°C AUTO-CLAVE CYCLE

$$P_{T2} = \frac{P_0 V_1 T_2}{V_2 T_1} + \text{Vapor pressure within the container}$$

where P_{T2} = internal pressure at 115°C (388°K); P_0 = assumed standard atmospheric pressure, 14.7 psia; T_1 = assumed temperature of liquid at time of filling, 20°C or 293°K; V_1 = Headspace volume at T_1 + Volume of H_2O in headspace at T_1 – Water vapor in air at T_1, and V_2 = Headspace volume at T_1 – Volume of liquid expansion at T_2.

For the syringes in question, headspace volume was calculated as 0.164 mL.

The volume of air in water at 20°C is known to be 18.7 mg/L; for a 0.5 mL fill volume, the volume is 9.35×10^{-3} mL.

Water vapor displacement of air at 20°C is known to be 1.9×10^{-2} mL/mL of headspace; therefore for a headspace volume of 0.164 = 3.25×10^{-3} mL.

Increase in volume of H_2O from 20°C to 115°C is known to be 5.37% (5.97% for an increase from 20°C to 121°C); therefore 0.5 mL fill volume will increase by 0.027 mL.

$$P_{115} = \frac{14.7 \times [0.164 + (9.35 \times 10^{-3}) - (3.25 \times 10^{-3})] \times 388}{293 \times (0.164 - 0.027)}$$
$$= 24.2 \text{ psia or } 1.67 \text{ bar}$$

Counterbalancing the internal pressure developing in filled syringes meeting the specifications given above would require an air overpressure of 1.67 bar above the pressure required to obtain 115°C during exposure (0.7 bar). The pressure during exposure would therefore be 2.4 bar (gauge).

ANNEX 2.   CALCULATING A SIMPLE F_0 VALUE

F_0 values can be calculated using Eq. (4.4):

$$F_0 = D_{121} (\log A - \log B)$$

where D_{121} = D-value of a heat-resistant microorganism at 121°C, say 1.5 min; A = number of microbiological contaminants per item, say 100; and B = SAL, usually 10^{-6}. Therefore

$$F_0 = 1.5(2 - [-6]) = 12 \text{ min.}$$

ANNEX 3. CALCULATING EQUIVALENT LETHALITY AT 134°C TO AN F_0 OF 11

The Parenteral Drug Association equation, Eq. (4.5), for calculating equivalent lethalities is

$$F^z{}_T = \frac{F^z{}_{121}}{L}$$

where $F^z{}_T$ = equivalent time at temperature T to achieve a specified lethality for contaminants with a specified z-value; $F^z{}_{121}$ = the equivalent time at 121°C to achieve the same lethality (when z equals 10°C, $F^z{}_{121} = F_0$); and L = lethal rate $(10[T - 121]/z)$.

$$F^z{}_{121} = F_0 = 11 \text{ min.}$$

$$L = \frac{10[134 - 121]}{10} = 10^{1.3} = 20^*$$

$$F^z{}_T = \frac{11}{20} = 0.55 \text{ min at } 134°C$$

$^*10^{1.3}$ is calculated by taking the logarithm of $10(\log_{10}$ of 10 is one) and multiplying by the power to which it is raised, in this case 1.3. The answer, 20 is the antilogarithm of 1.3.

Dry Heat Sterilization and Depyrogenation

Dry heat should be the method of choice for sterilization of heat-stable items that are damaged by moisture or are impervious to steam. It can in fact serve one or both of two functions; it may serve as a method of sterilization or as a method of sterilization and depyrogenation (destruction of bacterial endotoxins). Absence of bacterial endotoxins is a biological quality of equal or greater importance to sterility for pharmaceutical products and medical devices intended for parenteral application. None of the other large-scale methods of sterilization have the capability of destroying endotoxins and therefore depend to some extent on other processes for elimination of endotoxins prior to terminal sterilization.

Temperatures required for dry heat sterilization (over 160°C) are in a far higher range than those necessary for saturated steam sterilization (110 to 140°C). Depyrogenation requires even higher temperatures (200 to 400°C) if very long periods of exposure are to be avoided. Temperature/time combinations that are sufficient to meet requirements for endotoxin destruction are more than sufficient to sterilize the most highly contaminated items. Temperature/time combinations that are only sufficient to meet requirements of sterility are not sufficient to meet pharmacopoeial and regulatory requirements for endotoxin destruction.

Heat transfer from air to product items in dry heat processes is not efficient. The main mechanism is conduction; good insulators like air are by definition poor conductors.

I. EFFECTS OF DRY HEAT ON MICROORGANISMS AND BACTERIAL ENDOTOXINS

A. Inactivation of Microbial Populations

As with sterilization by saturated steam, thermal damage to biological systems as a result of dry heat sterilization processes is a function of absorbtion of heat energy. Inactivation of microorganisms is by oxidation. The kinetics of oxidation and population death approximate to first-order reactions, but they are significantly different from the processes of coagulation of cellular proteins found with moist heat sterilization in that they require far higher temperatures and proceed more slowly.

There are the usual species-to-species variations in response to dry heat. Spores are more resistant than vegetative cells. It does not follow that those microorganisms that are unusually resistant to moist heat sterilization processes are also resistant to dry heat conditions. Spores of *B. stearothermophilus* for instance are not as resistant to dry heat as spores of *Bacillus subtilis* var *niger*. This is exactly opposite to saturated steam. Numerous natural factors may protect spores against dry heat inactivation, notably antioxidants and reducing substances, which are capable of impeding the availability of oxygen to the oxidative site or target in the cell.

The terminology used in association with dry heat inactivation of microbial populations exactly parallels that of sterilization by saturated steam (see Chapter 4). The D_T-value is the time required to reduce a population to 10% of its initial numbers when held at a constant temperature T. The D-value of spores of *B. subtilis* var *niger* at 170°C (D_{170}) has been variously reported from around 8 s to 1.5 min for dry heat conditions.

The z-values for dry heat, i.e., the change in temperature required to effect a 10-fold change in D-value, are around 20°C, i.e., twice those normally quoted for saturated steam (10°C). Q_{10}-values of 1.6 have been quoted [1] for dry heat sterilization in the range 170 to 180°C, considerably lower than those quoted in Chapter 4 for saturated steam sterilization. This goes some way to justify the higher temperatures required from dry heat processes to meet the requirements of sterility.

B. Destruction of Bacterial Endotoxins (Pyrogens)

Pyrogens are substances that, when injected in sufficient amounts into the human or animal body, will cause a variety of symptoms of which the most recognizable is a rise in body temperature. They are therefore significant to sterile parenteral pharmaceuticals and to medical devices used for their administration. In pharmacopoeial terms, substances are categorized as pyrogenic or nonpyrogenic according to the response of injected rabbits versus specified temperature increases. The pharmacopoeial definition tends to be tautological but only reflects the limitations of the only analytical technology available at one time. Recent editions of the major pharmacopoeias are now recognizing an alternative to the rabbit pyrogen test. This is the LAL (*Limulus* amoebocyte lysate) test, a test specific for bacterial endotoxins.

There has been very little doubt for many years that by far the most significant source of pyrogens is microbiological. All microorganisms appear to be capable of producing pyrogens, and the most potent forms are associated with gram-negative bacteria.

All gram-negative bacteria are surrounded by a loosely structured envelope located externally to the peptidoglycan cell wall. Much of the enzymatic hydrolysis of nutrient macromolecules takes place within the cell envelope. The outer layer of the envelope is a permeability barrier effective against diffusion of exoenzymes into the greater environment; this outer layer is made up of lipopolysaccharides linked to phospholipids and proteins. The pyrogenic response has been shown to be stimulated by lipopolysaccharide fractions of the gram-negative cell envelope. These substances are termed bacterial endotoxins. Purified endotoxin is pyrogenic in lower doses than naturally occurring endotoxins in which the pyrogenicity is presumed to be modified by associated proteins and phospholipids. Bacterial endotoxity is not lost with loss of viability. Saturated steam, gamma radiation, and ethylene oxide sterilization processes that inactivate microorganisms are not capable of destroying bacterial endotoxins.

Purified endotoxin consists only of lipopolysaccharide. This itself has three distinct chemical regions; an inner core called lipid A, an intermediate polysaccharide layer, and an outer polysaccharide side chain. Lipid A, a highly substituted disaccharide of glucosamine, is responsible for pyrogenicity and other immunological and biological properties associated with endotoxin.

For most practical purposes the term endotoxin can be regarded as synonymous with pyrogen, depyrogenation with endotoxin destruction, and pyrogen-free with endotoxin-free.

Dry heat destruction of bacterial endotoxins is complex and poorly understood; much of the research data is contradictory [2]. Most experimental evidence has shown that destruction follows second-order chemical kinetics with a high initial rate of decrease of endotoxin followed by a much slower terminal rate. These second-order models give a better estimate of the kinetics of endotoxin destruction at temperatures above 250°C than in the 170 to 250°C temperature band. Impure endotoxin may account for these anomalies. There is practically no endotoxin destruction at temperatures below 80°C, and D-values for dry heat sterilization temperatures of around 170°C are as high as 20 min [2]. These observations are in agreement with published z-values of around 40°C for endotoxin destruction. Evidence of endotoxin destruction in practical situations is usually taken from empirical observation because of the uncertainty over its theoretical basis.

C. Other Methods of Bacterial Endotoxin Removal

Agents other than dry heat that have been shown to be capable of inactivating lipid A and hence eliminating the pyrogenicity of bacterial endotoxin include acid and alkaline hydrolysis, oxidation by hydrogen peroxide, and alkylation with strong alkylating agents (some depyrogenation can be expected to occur in ethylene oxide sterilization cycles). None of these methods is used on an industrial scale.

Removal of endotoxin from manufacturing equipment or materials can be done by appropriate washing and rinsing procedures. Pyrogen-free water can be obtained by several means. The oldest and most effective method is distillation —the heavyweight lipopolysaccharide molecules (MW of around 10^6) are left behind when water is rapidly boiled in a still. Reverse osmosis can remove 99.5 to 99.9% of water's endotoxin load in a single pass. For these reasons, distillation and reverse osmosis are the only two methods of preparing *Water for injection* allowed in the pharmacopoeias. The pharmacopoeial requirement for *Water for injection* is that there should be no more than 0.25 EU (endotoxin units)/mL.

Removal of endotoxin from low to medium molecular weight drugs and raw materials can be done by ultrafiltration, membrane filtration, depth filtration, or treatment with activated carbon [3]. These processes are complicated by the complex forms that can be adopted by bacterial endotoxin under differing circumstances. In its smallest form, bacterial endotoxin is likely to be lipopolysaccharide arranged in a micellar structure with hydrophilic side chains on the outside. Retention by hydrophobic membranes requires these aggregates to be broken up. These aggregates are retained on hydrophilic membranes with 0.025 μm pore size ratings but pass through 0.2 μm membranes.

D. Measurement of Bacterial Endotoxins (LAL Method)

In older editions of the pharmacopoeias, pharmaceutical products and medical devices could only be categorized as pyrogenic or nonpyrogenic by the *in vivo* rabbit test. This type of testing is being progressively replaced by an *in vitro* test specific for bacterial endotoxin. This is the LAL *(Limulus* amoebocyte lysate) test.

The LAL test depends upon a reaction between endotoxin and a "clottable" protein contained within the amoebocyte cells of the blood of the horseshoe crab *(Limulus polyphemus)*. The specificity of the reaction has been attributed [4] to a complex cascade of enzyme mediated reactions.

The "standard" LAL test is based on the formation of a semisolid gel between LAL and bacterial endotoxin and is conducted on the end-point principle. LAL reagent is supplied with an identified sensitivity, e.g., 0.03 endotoxin units (EU) per mL. This means that when mixed with an equal volume of the material under test a gel or clot will form if the material contains 0.03 EU/mL or greater. When it is necessary to quantify endotoxin concentration in a material it is usual to test a series of doubling dilutions against the reagent in temperature-controlled conditions. The greatest dilution that gives a positive (formation of a gel that withstands inversion of the reaction tube) is the end point, and the concentration of endotoxin in the material can be calculated by multiplying the dilution factor at the end point by the sensitivity of the LAL reagent.

Valid assays require careful internal standardization. The first USP batch of reference standard endotoxin (RSE) had a potency of 1 EU per 0.2 ng, but it is to the potency of RSE and not to weight that secondary standards (CSE, certified or calibrated standard endotoxin) are related. Within each series of end-point assays it is usual to set up a series of dilutions of CSE in concentrations of two times, equal to, half of, and one-fourth of the labelled claim of the LAL reagent being used. Valid assays require clotting from the two higher concentrations of CSE and absence of clotting from the two lower concentrations. A negative control and a positive control, in which the material under test is spiked with CSE at two times the labelled claim of the LAL reagent, are also required for each series of tests.

With doubling dilutions the accuracy of the method can be no better than plus or minus one twofold dilution; in other words, a derived value of 3 EU/mL should properly be reported as greater than 1.5 EU/mL but less than 6 EU/mL. When average values from replicate series are required, the exponential nature of the dilution series (i.e., 1:1, 1:2, 1:4, etc.) obliges the use of geometric means. Geometric means are calculated by multiplying the individual estimates and finding the nth root, thus

$$\sqrt[n]{a_1 \times a_2 \cdots \times a_n}$$

In practice this means determining the logarithm of each derived end point and dividing the sum of these by the number of end points. The geometric mean is the antilog of the mean log end point.

Other LAL methods are available based on turbidimetry and colorimetry. Reaction mixtures become turbid as gels, or clots form between LAL and bacterial endotoxin. Turbidimetry (sensitive to 0.001 EU/mL) is more sensitive for detecting bacterial endotoxin than gel clot assays (sensitive to 0.03 EU/mL) because turbidity is discernible at low concentrations of endotoxin at which firm gels do not form. The rate at which turbidity increases is proportional to the concentration of endotoxin in the material under test. This principle may be applied in end-point or kinetic assays.

With turbidimetric end-point assays, turbidity is measured after a fixed incubation period. By inclusion of standards alongside dilutions of the material under test, a standard curve can be created and the endotoxin concentration can be read off this curve for the material under test. Equipment using microtiter plates is commercially available to minimize the amounts of LAL reagent necessary and to maximize the number of test sets per set of standards. The period of incubation over which turbidimetric end-point assays is conducted is critical. All samples will be equally turbid with overlong incubation; if incubation times are too short none of the samples will be measurably turbid. It is not possible to stop the reaction to take the readings.

The turbidimetric principle and automated microtiter plate reading apparatus are more commonly used in the kinetic rather than the end-point mode. Turbidity readings of each reaction mixture are taken at frequent intervals throughout an incubation period. The logarithm of the time (the onset time) taken to reach a specified level of turbidity is inversely proportional and linearly related to the logarithm of the concentration of endotoxin in the material under test. Standardization is necessary with each series of assays. This approach is only practical for routine application using microprocessor-controlled equipment.

Chromogenic methods rely on the fact that there are enzymatic reactions within the process of gel formation. Gel formation in simplest terms is a two-stage process. First there is the activation of a previously inactive clotting enzyme by reaction with endotoxin, and second there is the formation of a clot by a reaction between the activated enzyme and a coagulen substrate. In chromogenic methods the coagulen substrate is replaced by a synthetic analog containing a chromophore. When attached to the synthetic substrate the chromophore is colorless, but when cleaved by the activated clotting enzyme it turns yellow. The rate of color production is proportional to the concentration of bacterial endotoxin in the material under test. The reaction is pH sensitive and can be stopped by addition of acid.

The methods of chromogenic LAL testing are very similar to those for turbidimetric LAL testing. Their advantages over gel clot and turbidimetric methods are in relation to the range of products with which they can be used. In all
three methods, there are broadly two stages that are potentially subject to interference or inhibition from the material under test. The first is the activation of
the clotting enzyme by reaction with endotoxin; this is common to all three
methods because it is this reaction that is specific for endotoxin. The second
stage of the methods has only to do with the development of the first-stage reaction such that the progress of the first-stage reaction can be detected and monitored. The second stage reactions involved in the formation of the three-dimensional matrix of the gel upon which gel clot and turbidimetric assays are based
are far more complex and therefore far more subject to interference than the
comparatively simple cleaving of the chromophore in the chromogenic methods.

II. APPLICATIONS OF DRY HEAT STERILIZATION

Dry heat sterilization is available as both large-scale and small-scale processes.
Oven sterilization of laboratory equipment and medical instruments is often the
most reliable and economic method regardless of scale but is usually found in
laboratory-scale and hospital-scale operations. Larger-scale industrial ovens are
used in pharmaceutical manufacture, more often in association with sterilization
of intermediates than with sterilization of finished products, for instance, the
bulk sterilization of petrolatum bases for sterile (mainly ophthalmic) ointments
and sterilization of powdered excipients in shallow trays (e.g., sodium citrate) for
subsequent aseptic blending. The larger-scale processes usually operate to sterilize only, because the higher temperatures required for the dual steriliza-
tion/depyrogenation function would be prohibitively long.

Dry heat tunnel sterilizers are only found in large-scale processes. Their
main application is in the sterilization and depyrogenation of glass primary
product-contact containers (bottles, ampoules, vials) prior to aseptic filling and
sealing.

A. Ovens and Tunnels

Sterilizing ovens are not intrinsically complicated. Figure 1 is a diagrammatic
representation of a fairly typical sterilizing oven. HEPA-filtered air (see Chapter
8) is heated by passage over electric heating elements; heat is transferred from
the air to the product by forced convection.

There are four stages involved in oven sterilization. They are (a) drying,
(b) heat-up, (c) exposure, and (d) cool-down.

In the drying stage, moisture is driven off the product to the atmosphere
until the air temperature in the oven is approximately 80°C, at which point a baf-

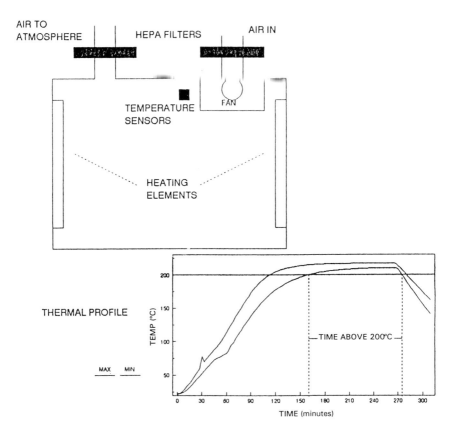

Fig. 1 Typical sterilizing oven.

fle closes to allow the temperature within the sealed oven to reach its operating level. A positive pressure is maintained within the oven throughout the cycle.

Exposure is timed from the moment the sterilization thermal sensor located near the top of the oven reaches the set temperature. At the end of the timed exposure period the heating elements are switched off and cool-down begins. In some ovens, cooling may be accelerated by forced passage of cold HEPA-filtered air over the product during the cool-down phase.

Each stage of oven sterilization has some considerable drawbacks associated with intrinsic low heat transfer rates from air to product. Inevitably this means slow heating up and cooling down, a problem that can extend cycles from a nominal 2 h to more than 3 h for practical purposes. A second drawback has to do with lack of uniformity of temperature within the oven. Hot air has a tendency to stratify and to penetrate only poorly around masses of cooler materials.

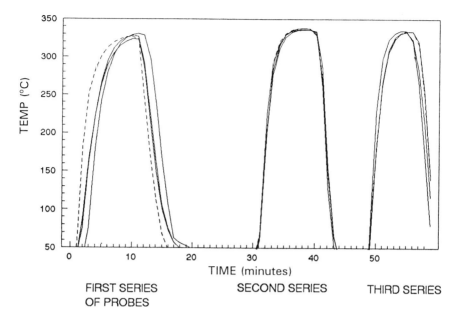

Fig. 2 Thermal profiles through LAF tunnel (progressive).

Compensating for these difficulties often forces the actual operating temperatures of oven sterilization processes to considerably higher levels than the nominal temperature. The potential for heat damage and even charring of the materials being sterilized from a combination of these drawbacks needs no further elaboration.

Dry heat tunnel sterilization is a continuous process in contrast to the batch processes in ovens. Sterilization and depyrogenation in tunnels exemplifies the additive nature of thermal processes; for most of the time spent in the tunnel the product is being subjected to rising temperatures (Fig. 2) rather than being held at a constantly maintained exposure temperature. The temperature of the tunnel is held constant, with the temperature of the product changing as it proceeds through. Energy is not being lost to heating and reheating between cycles as it is with ovens.

Figure 3 is a roughly to scale comparison of the two main types of sterilizing tunnel in industrial use, radiant-heat sterilizing tunnels and the more recently developed laminar airflow (LAF) tunnel sterilizers.

Radiant-heat sterilizing tunnels have had extremely wide usage in pharmaceutical manufacture. Infrared heaters, located in the roof of the tunnel, heat surfaces of product items passing through the tunnel and internal surfaces of the tunnel itself. The heat is then disseminated throughout the product items by

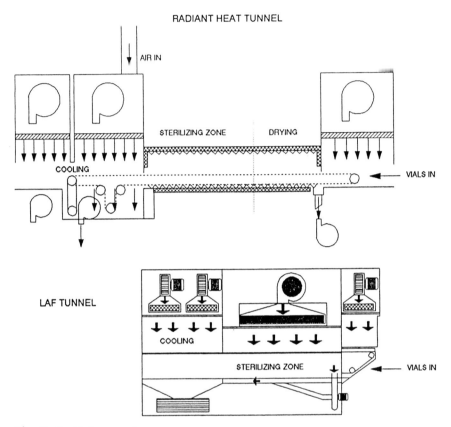

Fig. 3 Sterilizing tunnels.

radiation, conduction, and turbulent airflow. They are, however, quite large, belt speeds are slow, product heat-up may be less than uniform, and they may create particulate problems. That is not to say that these problems cannot be controlled.

Excessive numbers of particles may be generated in radiant-heat sterilizing tunnels from deterioration of the heating elements and the moving belt, and from abrasion between moving product items. Particles are not generally effectively removable from this type of tunnel, although performance can be improved by installation of HEPA filters at the tunnel entrance and at its junction with the cooling zone. It is of course quite standard to find the cooling zone equipped with HEPA filters to protect the sterility of the items that have passed through the tunnel en route to an aseptic filling room.

In LAF tunnels air is heated by passage over heating elements prior to HEPA filtration, so at least one source (deterioration of the elements) is excluded from the sterilizer at source. The sweeping action of the laminar airflow then contributes to the removal of other particles generated within the tunnel. Heat transfer is also much faster, contributing to a lower risk of product contamination from particles purely as a result of shorter throughput times (around 50% of the throughput time expected from radiant-heat tunnels).

III. TEMPERATURE/TIME CRITERIA FOR STERILIZATION AND DEPYROGENATION

Sterilization temperature/time combinations for dry heat are directly analogous to those for sterilization by saturated steam. The options are compendial cycles, overkill, or a validated 10^{-6} sterility assurance level (SAL). The USP is curiously ambiguous about SALs for dry heat processes; although accepting 10^{-6} as a standard it stresses that the approach is often to achieve SALs of 10^{-12}. This is because so many dry heat sterilization treatments are also intended to inactivate bacterial endotoxins (see below).

Compendial cycles are only applicable to ovens because there are too many variables in tunnels (belt speeds, stoppages, preceding materials, etc.) to be encompassed in simple generalized process specifications. Compendial cycles in the *British Pharmacopoeia* require 160°C for 2 hs, 170°C for 1 h, or 180°C for 30 min. The USP refers rather obliquely to temperatures in excess of 250°C.

In the absence of precise knowledge of the dry heat inactivation characteristics of the actual microbiogical contaminants of the product, the reference microorganisms for overkill (twelve D-values) and SAL targets are spores of *B. subtilis* var *niger*. A D_{170}-value of at least 1.5 min may be assumed for these spores. For dry heat temperatures other than 170°C, there is a concept comparable to the F_0 concept for steam sterilization. It is termed the F_H concept and references lethality to equivalent times at 170°C. The units of F_H-value are minutes or seconds. Calculations of F_H use the same equations as calculations of F_0, but the z-value of 20°C is substituted in the case of dry heat.

Consider the BP compendial cycle of 170°C for 1 h versus a D_{170}-value of 1.5 min for spores of *B. subtilis* var *niger*. Clearly some forty D-values are obtainable exclusive of the lethal input during heat-up and cool-down. This is far in excess of the twelve D-values necessary to claim overkill and would permit a 10^{-6} SAL to be obtained for items contaminated by up to 10^{34} colony-forming units prior to sterilization. The F_H values of the other two compendial cycles are 95 min for the 180°C cycle and 38 min for the 60°C cycle—all far in excess of the minimum necessary.

There are no compendial cycles recommended for endotoxin reduction. The standard quoted in the USP and being enforced by the FDA is that a claim to depyrogenation should be supported by evidence that endotoxin present on the product prior to treatment has been inactivated to no more than 1/1000 of the original amount (three $\log_{10}$ reductions). The minimum time required to obtain three $\log_{10}$ reductions of endotoxin at 170°C has been variously reported to be from 3 h to over 66 h. Six $\log_{10}$ reductions have been demonstrated at 250°C. In summary, depyrogenation cycles have to be developed and validated empirically. However, the USP recommends a temperature of at least 250°. Considering that the F_H value of a 5-min cycle at 250°C (regardless of any heat-up or cool-down lethality) is an unbelievably long time, it is safe to assume that any dry heat cycle that achieves depyrogenation will more than achieve any contemporary sterility assurance standard.

IV. VALIDATION AND ROUTINE CONTROL OF DRY HEAT STERILIZATION

A. Validation

Beyond the usual engineering aspects of validation with regard to specification, installation, commissioning, qualification, and calibration, the two important aspects of validation of dry heat processes are thermal validation and endotoxin validation. Biological studies with spores of *B. subtilis* var *niger* are rarely necessary.

The purpose of thermal validation is to demonstrate that heat is uniformly delivered to all parts of the oven or tunnel load. With ovens the principles are exactly the same as for autoclaves. The exercise of thermal validation of tunnels is usually more complicated due to having to place thermocouples in product items, which are then allowed to be carried on the moving belt through the tunnel. The difficulties however are not insurmountable. The lowest temperatures in the load should be determined rigorously from one side of the tunnel to the other, from the leading edge of a new load of product items to the trailing edge. It is important that the coldest spots be identified for subsequent endotoxin inactivation studies.

For endotoxin destruction, items must be spiked with bacterial endotoxin and passed through preferably shortened (for tunnels this means faster belt speeds than specified) or cooler cycles than the proposed process specification. The spiked items should be placed in previously identified cold spots. They are then retrieved and assayed by the LAL method for remaining traces of endotoxin. The key to doing this successfully is to be sure that each item is spiked with at least 1000 times as much endotoxin as the minimal quantity detectable by the available recovery and assay techniques.

B. Routine Control

Routine control of ovens should be by temperature and time. A floating probe should be placed in the load and recognized as the critical measure. Forced air fans and over-pressurization systems should be equipped with fail-safe warning systems to ensure their continuing function.

Tunnels require the belt speed to be specified and controlled. When linked with other fixed-speed equipment such as washers and fillers, changes in tunnel belt speed often become self-evident. Temperature monitoring should reflect the coolest zone in the tunnel and include a reference sensor related to the temperature conditions recorded in the product during validation. Floating probes in the product are not usual (for reasons of practicality).

Routine use of biological indicators is not necessary. Routine endotoxin controls using spiked samples have never been seriously proposed.

REFERENCES

1. Ernst, R. R. (1977). Sterilization by heat. In *Disinfection, Sterilization and Preservation* (S. S. Block, ed.). Philadelphia: Lea and Febiger.
2. Ludwig, J. D., and Avis, K. E. (1990). Dry heat inactivation of endotoxin on the surface of glass. *Journal of Parenteral Science and Technology* **44**: 4–12.
3. Weary, M., and Pearson, F. (1988). A manufacturer's guide to depyrogenation. *Biopharm* (April 1988): 22–29.
4. Dawson, M. (1992). Endotoxin testing of medical devices. In *Bioburden in Medical Devices and Surgical Dressing Manufacture*. Proceedings of a EUCOMED Conference, March 23/24, 1992. Brussels, Belgium: EUCOMED.

6
Sterilization by Ethylene Oxide

Of the several methods of sterilization that rely on inactivation of microorganisms to meet their objective, sterilization by exposure to ethylene oxide is by far the most difficult to control. The main advantages of ethylene oxide as a sterilant do not lie in speed, simplicity, or reliability of control but rather in the range of materials that can withstand treatment without damage. It is not used for pharmaceuticals. It is, however, an extensively used alternative to irradiation as a method of cold sterilization for heat-labile medical devices and pharmaceutical packaging components. Industrial-scale and laboratory-scale technologies are available.

Ethylene oxide is a cyclic ether (C_2H_4O) with a boiling point of $10.7°C$ at atmospheric pressure. It is colorless and virtually odorless. In its pure form ethylene oxide is highly flammable in air; in particular circumstances it may be explosive. Its first practical application as a biocide was as recently as the 1940s when it began to be used for disinfestation of food crops. It is still used to reduce the microbial contamination of bulk spices. As with gamma radiation, its development as a sterilization process for medical devices went hand in hand with the increased availability of biologically inert plastics. Until radiation sterilization became competitive in the 1960s and 1970s, it was the single most important method of industrial-scale cold sterilization. In terms of volume of items sterilized it has now been overtaken by irradiation, partly because of simple economic reasons and partly because it has been found to be carcinogenic.

I. INACTIVATION EFFECTS ON MICROORGANISMS AND MICROBIAL POPULATIONS

Inactivation and death of microorganisms results from alkylating effects on sulfhydryl, amino, carboxyl, and hydroxyl groups within the cell. Ethylene oxide replaces labile hydrogen atoms in these groups. Lethal effects are through blockage of reactive sites on metabolically active molecules. Comparison of activation energies has shown that DNA and RNA are the most likely target molecules. Unlike most other chemical sterilants, which are several thousand times more active against vegetative cells than spores, the resistance of spores to ethylene oxide and other alkylating agents is less than ten times greater than the resistance of vegetative organisms. For instance, spores of *Bacillus stearothermophilus* and *Clostridium sporogenes* have been shown to show a very similar response to vegetative cells of *Streptoccus faecium* when exposed under identical conditions [1].

The kinetics of inactivation of microbial populations exposed to ethylene oxide are exponential [2] when the logarithm of the number of survivors is plotted against time with all other factors (e.g., gas concentration, humidity, temperature) held constant. Shouldered curves have been occasionally noted; instances of "tailed" inactivation kinetics have been ascribed to clumping or environmental protection. Good experimental data are not easily obtained. Experimental design should concentrate on rapid attainment of the gas concentration intended. Inactivation from residual sterilant may also lead to misleading results.

D-values have only a very limited value for comparing the resistance of various microorganisms and various ethylene oxide processes. This is because inactivation characteristics are subject to the influence of numerous other variables that are unavoidably part of ethylene oxide sterilization technology. The complexity of interaction between gas concentration, temperature of exposure, humidity during exposure, pressure during exposure, and the condition of the microbial population prior to exposure has not been adequately described by theory.

A. Effects of Gas Concentration on Microbial Response to Ethylene Oxide

The effects of the concentration of ethylene oxide on inactivation of microorganisms are quite straightforward. Within limiting concentrations, the effect of doubling the gas concentration doubles the rate of inactivation. Concentrations of less than 300 mg/L are insufficient to achieve sterility within practical process times. Very high gas concentrations imply very high pressures, and the gas laws dictate that an increase in temperature is necessary within a sterilizer at constant volume to maintain equilibrium conditions at increased pressures, possibly too high a temperature to meet the intended cold sterilization purposes. In practice, gas concentrations are usually within a range of 500 to 800 mg/L, which is a practical compromise among sterilization effectiveness and process time and for the constraints imposed by available technology.

B. Effects of Temperature on Microbial Response to Ethylene Oxide

Alkylation reactions respond to temperature in the same way as normal chemical reactions. Under constant conditions and within the range of limiting gas concentrations, ethylene oxide sterilization follows first-order chemical kinetics, i.e., the rate of inactivation is approximately doubled (the D-value is halved) for every 10°C rise in temperature. The lowest temperature at which ethylene oxide sterilization is theoretically possible is the temperature at which the gas liquefies, which is 10.7°C at atmospheric pressure. Upper limits of temperature are of less importance, because the whole point of using ethylene oxide is to achieve cold sterilization. Other restricting factors at high temperatures are polymerization and the pressure rating of ethylene oxide sterilizers. Industrial-scale processes normally operate within a cold sterilization range of 50 to 60°C.

C. Effects of Humidity on Microbial Response to Ethylene Oxide

Humidity is the single most important factor influencing the effects of ethylene oxide on microbial populations. Ethylene oxide is quite simply ineffective against dehydrated microorganisms in a dry environment.

Ethylene oxide is a chemical sterilant and must therefore come into contact with target molecules (DNA and RNA) that are physically located within the "heart" of the cell, or within the core of bacterial spores. Water acts as a carrier of ethylene oxide through permeable barriers. The water activity of the microbial cell and the relative humidity of the environment in which it finds itself are of critical importance to water movement and to the penetration of chemical sterilants to their target sites. The situation becomes complex when it is understood that ethylene oxide can itself increase the permeation of water through permeable barriers.

Most experimental work on the effects of humidity has been done on bacterial spores. Bacterial spores can survive over a greater range of water activities and moisture contents than vegetative cells. In particular they can withstand considerable degrees of desiccation. Although spores are not actively dividing microorganisms, they are not completely metabolically inactive. Ernst and Doyle [3] postulated that dynamic equilibria exist between spores and their immediate environment, determined in the main by the number and types of active sites on the surfaces of the spores. Active sites become physically withdrawn from the surfaces as the spores dehydrate. Spores with higher moisture contents and therefore greater numbers of exposed active sites exhibit higher rates of exchange of molecules with their immediate environment than do dry spores with low water activities.

The equilibrium between the spore and the environment can operate in two directions, i.e., with water moving predominantly from the environment into the spore or conversely predominantly out of the spore into the environment. The direction of the equilibrium as it affects water movement is for the most part a function of the relative humidity of the environment. With relatively high environmental moisture, water will move into the spore. The concentration gradient between the moisture content of the spore and the moisture content of the environment acts as a driving force in accord with Fick's laws of diffusion. At low environmental relative humidities water will move out of the spore into the environment.

The significance of this model is that it describes the optimal situation for water permeation into the spore and therefore ethylene oxide permeation to its target site as a function of the moisture content of the spore and the relative humidity of the environment during exposure. The rate of microbial inactivation therefore increases (as long as all other factors are held constant) with increased relative humidity during exposure. Kaye and Phillips [4] demonstrated a 33% RH optimum for microbial inactivation as a result of exposure to ethylene oxide. In practical situations it is better to err on the side of too much rather than too little moisture. With industrial-scale ethylene oxide sterilization, humidity levels are usually in the range of 50% to 60% RH. The upper limit is usually dictated by deleterious effects on packaging.

D. Other Factors Affecting Microbial Response to Ethylene Oxide

Any factor that prevents permeation of ethylene oxide to its target sites within the cell is capable of adversely influencing the rate of inactivation. Such factors may include organic matter or inorganic crystalline material. Reduced sterilant penetration has also been noted with clumped cells. These effects are probably due as much to physical factors as to chemical ones. Although ethylene oxide has a history of use as a crude fumigant, it is suitable as a sterilant only for clean items, which components for pharmaceutical products and medical devices can always be supposed to be when manufactured according to the Good Manufacturing Practices.

Dadd and Daley [5] observed that some microorganisms may have a limited ability to overcome the effects of ethylene oxide but that this did not to any great extent confer resistance. The spore coat did not contribute to the resistance of resistant bacterial spores except as it constituted an increased number of alternative target sites for alkylation. Spores did not become as sensitive to ethylene oxide as vegetative cells until they had fully emerged from inside their spore coats.

II. APPLICATIONS OF ETHYLENE OXIDE STERILIZATION

Ethylene oxide sterilization is suitable for both small-scale and large-scale applications. It is primarily a method of cold sterilization and has so many associated complications that it is never used in preference to thermal sterilization for heat-stable materials. Sterilization by gamma radiation is more reliable than ethylene oxide for cold sterilization, and it is simpler to control. It is, however, limited by suitability of materials and only operates on a large scale.

Ethylene oxide is penetrative (but less penetrative than gamma radiation). On an industrial scale this allows devices sealed within primary containers to be packed into shelf packs or shippers and palletized before sterilization. Product is normally sterilized on pallets.

In order to inactivate microorganisms, ethylene oxide must come into contact with target sites in the microbial cell. Even though ethylene oxide is very penetrative, this is a major complicating factor for any method of terminal sterilization. Free movement of the gas to all parts and internal cavities of each item being sterilized is an essential prerequisite of the process. This imposes certain constraints (arguably restrictive constraints in the case of individually packed single-use medical devices) on the design of product items, the design of packaging materials, the choice of packaging materials, and the manner in which products are packed in boxes, stacked, palletized, and loaded into sterilizers.

A basic prerequisite of product design is that sealed internal cavities should be avoided for products intended for terminal sterilization by exposure to ethylene oxide. Disposable hypodermic syringes were among the first medical devices to be sterilized in large numbers by ethylene oxide. Syringe plungers are usually fitted with elastomeric tips that seal with an interference fit to the internal barrel wall at two diameters separated by an internal cavity (Fig. 1). The

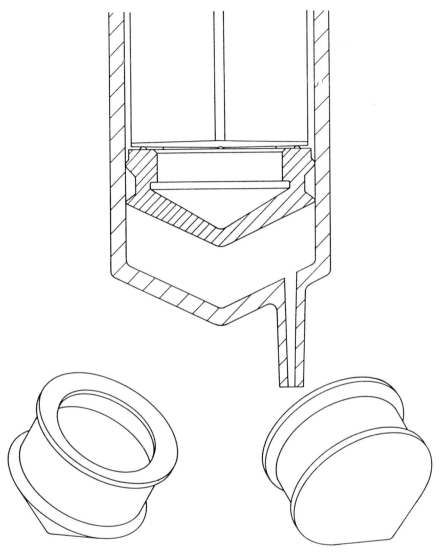

Fig. 1 Internal cavities in hypodermic syringes.

region between the two "lands" of the plunger tip is usually considered the most difficult to sterilize because of uncertainty concerning gas penetration. Although this region is strictly a sealed cavity, ethylene oxide may gain access if the plunger tip is made from a gas-permeable material. While natural rubber remains the commonest material for manufacture of plunger tips, the ready absorption of ethylene oxide into this material prevents poor penetration from restricting gaseous sterilization of syringes. However, other elastomeric materials, which may not be as permeable to ethylene oxide, are becoming competitive with rubber and are beginning to offer advantages in the areas of materials costs and consistency of quality.

Penetration is important to the selection of packaging materials where these are the primary barrier to microbiological contamination of the device after sterilization and before use. Most often, cold-sterilized medical devices are packed in flexible rather than rigid primary containers. Permeable materials are necessary when ethylene oxide is the method of sterilization. Paper is commonly used because it has a history of successful usage, because the technology for printing on paper is readily available, and because it is cheap and recyclable. On the other hand, it is not always impermeable to microorganisms; it is opaque, and it may tear easily on devices with sharp edges or when subjected to pressure differentials or when carelessly handled or transported. Alternative permeable materials that avoid the disadvantages of paper, such as spun-bonded polyolefins (Tyvek), are very expensive. Almost any material can be sealed to any other material, and therefore composite packs made from more than one material are common. One part of the pack may be gas permeable, the other impermeable, one part opaque and printable, the other transparent. The technology of ethylene oxide sterilization involves high humidities and pressure changes. The potentially deleterious effects of these aspects of the sterilization processes on seal integrity are not insignificant.

With some other medical devices, only the sterility of the internal lumina (fluid path sterility) is being claimed. Typically these devices are sealed and self-contained without any primary packaging. Some drug delivery systems, for instance, are sealed at their ends, and fluid path sterility only is being claimed. Self-contained sterile insulin syringes are one of the largest bulk volume sterile medical devices in the world. With these devices it is necessary to vent the caps or seals to allow access of ethylene oxide. This creates a clear conflict with the requirement for hermetic sealing of the sterilized device against entry of microorganisms.

One way of resolving this has been to ensure that any venting is achieved only through sterilant-permeable antimicrobial filters. Alternatively, vent caps may be designed to have a small unfiltered tortuous passage to the exterior that can be demonstrated empirically to make entry of the microorganisms into the fluid path improbable. Before adopting such designs, manufacturers should address the choice of ethylene oxide versus other methods of cold sterilization. With radiation sterilization, for instance, venting is not necessary.

III. ETHYLENE OXIDE STERILIZATION PROCESSES

Ethylene oxide is a product of the petroleum industry primarily produced as a starting material for polyethylene glycol (antifreeze) and other related substances. For sterilization purposes it is commercially available in the pure form or as mixtures with fluorinated hydrocarbons or carbon dioxide. Pure ethylene oxide is highly flammable in air. In sterilization it is normally used in conjunction with an inert gas such or carbon dioxide or nitrogen from a separate source. Commercially available gas mixtures are nonflammable under normal operating conditions of temperature and pressure. Mixtures of 12% ethylene oxide : 88% dichlorodifluoromethane, and 20% ethylene oxide : 80% carbon dioxide have been commonly used. Environmental issues relating to the use of fluorinated hydrocarbons are seriously restricting the use of so-called 12:88.

Pure ethylene oxide is cheaper than gas mixtures. At one time it was used undiluted, but it is no longer possible to have this practice underwritten for insurance purposes. All existing processes, whether using pure ethylene oxide plus a diluent or using a gas mixture, operate at a positive pressure to the atmosphere. Any leakage of gas from the chamber must therefore be toward dilution in the external environment rather than toward formation of an explosive mixture in the chamber. Gas mixtures with fluorinated hydrocarbons or carbon dioxide require higher operating pressures to achieve the same sterilant concentrations as diluted pure ethylene oxide systems.

Industrial-scale ethylene oxide sterilization usually takes place in steel pressure vessels (Fig. 2) equipped with water or steam jackets to maintain the operating temperature within reasonable tolerances throughout the sterilization process or cycle. Intrinsically the equipment is no more elaborate than that used for steam sterilization except that the vessels are often considerably larger. Ethylene oxide sterilizers with capacities of greater than 1,000 ft^3 (eight or ten pallets) are not uncommon. Essential features include some means of evacuating the chamber to facilitate the introduction of ethylene oxide and steam, and some means of vaporizing (usually a heat exchanger) the ethylene oxide that exists in its liquid phase in pressurized cylinders or drums.

Pure ethylene oxide for use in conjunction with a diluent gas and 20:80 mixtures of ethylene oxide are potentially explosive; all electrical equipment, switchgear, and monitoring and measuring systems used in association with these forms of the sterilant must be sparkproof. Serious consideration should be given to the location and design of gas stores and sterilization suites in relation to other areas within a factory, in relation to other factory buildings, and in relation to the local community. Blow-out roofs, windows, and walls are commonly installed with the intention of channelling the shock waves from an explosion in the direction of least harm.

The internal construction of ethylene oxide sterilizers is uncomplicated and uncluttered. There may be some form of forced air circulation to prevent stratification of the various types of gas present in the chamber during sterilization (sterilant, diluent, moisture). There should be the devices or sample ports for continuous monitoring and recording of temperature and pressure within the

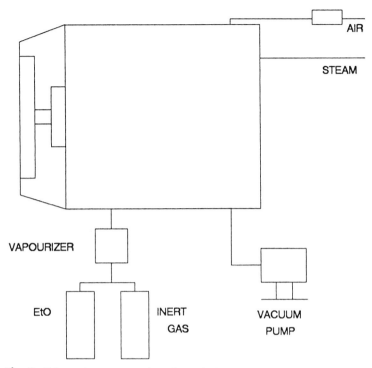

Fig. 2 Schematic representation of a typical ethylene oxide sterilizer.

chamber. There may be associated equipment to monitor gas concentration. All electrical equipment used in association with pure ethylene oxide sterilizers must be sparkproofed.

In some instances there may be an ancillary chamber in which the product load is equilibrated to a specified temperature and humidity prior to its introduction into the sterilizer. The intentions of preconditioning are threefold:

(a) To equilibrate the microorganisms contaminating the product to conditions of temperature and water activity that are optimal for their inactivation by exposure to ethylene oxide.

(b) To equilibrate the packaging (primarily cellulosic materials) to the conditions of the sterilizer in order to prevent deleterious equilibria arising in the sterilization chamber.

(c) To optimize the utilization of the sterilizer. If equilibration is not done elsewhere it must be done in the sterilizer. The residence time of the product in the sterilizer must then be longer than it need be. Preconditioning chambers that do not operate under pressure are cheaper to build and to operate than sterilizers.

It is critical to ensure that the length of time between the removal of a load from the preconditioning chamber and the beginning of its sterilization cycle is rigorously controlled. It is all too easy, particularly in dry climates with very low humidities, for equilibrium to be rapidly lost.

A typical sterilization cycle (Fig. 3) begins with evacuation of the loaded sterilizer to a predetermined level. It is most important that sufficient vacuum is achieved, not only because it may affect the settings for subsequent phases of the process but also because adequate air removal must be assured to avoid the formation of explosive mixtures with oxygen.

A known amount of steam is then introduced and the sterilizer is left to "soak" for a short period. This is followed by injection of the sterilizing gas to its specified pressure. The sterilizer and its contents are then held under these conditions for the specified time of exposure. At the end of this period the gas is removed by evacuation and replaced by air that has passed through a bacteria-retentive filter.

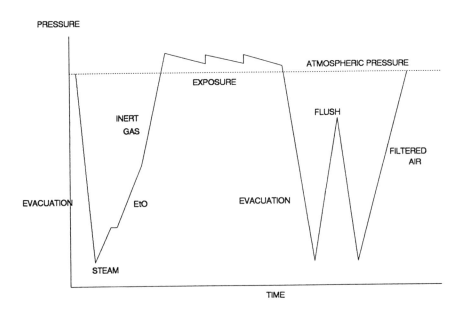

Fig. 3 Typical ethylene oxide sterilization cycle.

In routine sterilization, gas concentrations of 500–800 mg/L, temperatures of 50–60°C, and relative humidities of at least 50% RH are used. The pressure within the sterilizer is important only as it relates to obtaining adequate ethylene oxide concentration as dictated by the gas mixture being used. These operating criteria are as much a function of the technology of the process as they are a reflection of the optimal conditions for sterilization. To a great extent, the gas concentrations, temperatures, and relative humidities used for ethylene oxide sterilization are dictated by the relationships that govern the pressure and temperature of gases at fixed volumes. At temperatures lower than 50°C there may be difficulty in maintaining the vapor state of the gases in the chamber. Higher gas concentrations achieved through increased pressure may result in condensation of water or ethylene oxide unless accompanied by increasing temperature.

The most important phase of the sterilization cycle is the introduction of steam under vacuum. Initial evacuation of the sterilizer is completely unavoidable. It is also potentially deleterious to microbial inactivation. During evacuation the load in the sterilizer loses heat, and more importantly it loses moisture. Steam injection restores the temperature and moisture content of the load to its correct equilibrium. This must be achieved before the sterilant gas is added. There are two main reasons for this:

(a) Ethylene oxide has a greater capacity to penetrate through materials than water has. If the two substances were to be injected into a sterilizer at the same time, the ethylene oxide molecules would permeate and diffuse through the load fastest, leaving the water molecules behind. Ethylene oxide is a comparatively poor sterilant in the absence of moisture.

(b) Water reacts with ethylene oxide. If the two substances were to be injected at the same time, the effective concentration of both systems would be reduced. This would have a deleterious effect on the rate of microbial inactivation.

IV. VALIDATION AND ROUTINE CONTROL OF ETHYLENE OXIDE STERILIZATION

Sterilization by exposure to ethylene oxide is bounded by at least four variables: gas concentration, time of exposure, temperature, and humidity. It is also affected by product design, packaging design, and the composition of packaging materials. The shape, size, and materials of construction of individual sterilizers, the location of gas entry ports, and the presence or absence of forced circulation may all influence sterility assurance. There is no theory to describe these interactions. Validation and routine control of ethylene oxide sterilization processes boils down finally to the integration of all of these variables by reference to biological monitors.

Before validation even, very serious consideration must be given to the nature of the product that is intended to be sterilized and the type of packaging it is to be presented in. Again, it is only experience and experiment that can indicate and confirm the suitability of particular presentations for ethylene oxide sterilization.

Most of the product-related factors need only be evaluated on a broad basis; products compatible with one ethylene oxide sterilization process are generally compatible with most others. Some of the factors that ought to be addressed include

(a) Choice of materials. Although ethylene oxide is probably compatible with a wider range of materials than any other major sterilization process, the choice of materials is not without pitfalls. Some polymers show signs of chemical degradation as a result of chemical reaction during sterilization. Some polymers craze in response to gas mixtures containing fluorinated hydrocarbons but are satisfactory for other ethylene oxide processes. Physical properties may alter, and dimensional tolerances may be changed through shrinkage or expansion. Materials should be chosen to allow degassing (aeration) in a reasonable time frame.

(b) Product design. The product must be designed with the consideration that the sterilant must be able to penetrate to all parts. Functional tolerances should allow for the intense (and often abrupt) pressure and temperature changes that arise in ethylene oxide sterilization.

Consideration of packaging materials should be specific to particular sterilization cycles and should extend beyond primary packaging materials to include the potential effects of secondary packaging (shelf packs or shippers) and pallets on sterility assurance. In some instances these latter factors may need to be addressed on a sterilizer-specific basis, where variations have been suspected of being the cause of erratic and unpredictable biological test failures. The important packaging factors to consider are

(a) Choice of materials. There is a wide variety of materials available for primary packaging (i.e., the packaging that is intended to provide the hermetic environment for the sterilized product) of ethylene oxide sterilizable medical devices. The permeability of the pack to ethylene oxide and water vapor is of utmost importance, but this does not mean that the complete pack has to be made from permeable materials. The pack must be able to withstand pressure changes without materials rupture. This may often lead to composite packs made from permeable and nonpermeable webs; other considerations, for instance price, "printability," and appearance, account for the large number of composite packs currently being sterilized.

Secondary packaging materials are usually made from corrugated cardboard; the grade and the direction of fluting can have serious effects on sterility assurance and on sterility maintenance. Absorption of moisture in secondary packaging may divert the availability of ethylene oxide from its target sites. Insufficient structural rigidity of secondary packaging may lead to damage to primary packaging during or after sterilization with consequent loss of sterility.

(b) Seals. Primary packs must be sealed in a manner that will prevent microbiological ingress, withstand the rigors of the sterilization cycle, and still be easily openable by the customer at point of use. Within some packs there may be more than one type of seal, some intended to be opened, others intended to be permanently closed. Syringe packs usually direct the user to the openable seal by a printed instruction. Often this is disregarded in clinical practice, where users have found it easier to burst the packets open. The characteristics of good microbiological seals and of equipment that is capable of producing consistent seal quality can only be evaluated empirically.

A. Validation of Ethylene Oxide Sterilization Processes

The overall scheme of validation of ethylene oxide sterilization is no different from validation of any other process. With new equipment it requires careful consideration of design before specification (Design Qualification), confirmation that received equipment conforms to its specification (Installation Qualification), and confirmation that received equipment can perform its specified functions when assembled, plumbed in, and linked up to local services (Operational Qualification).

Process qualification of ethylene oxide sterilization is both sterilizer specific and product specific. It is particularly directed toward the measurable parameters of the whole sterilization cycle. If external preconditioning is used, validation should address the measurable parameters of all combinations of preconditioning chamber and sterilizer. Where one preconditioning chamber may serve two or more sterilizers, or where one sterilizer may be served by two or more preconditioning chambers, cycle-to-cycle variability should be minimal. The essence of successful ethylene oxide sterilization lies in the establishment of a complete process specification with very tight tolerances. The integral effects of the specified conditions on assurance of sterility can only be validated by reference to biological monitors.

1. Load Specification: The product and its primary and secondary packaging must be specified. The loading pattern of primary packs into shelf packs should be specified. Occlusion of gas-permeable surfaces one against the other should be avoided if sterility is to be assured.

The loading pattern of shelf packs on pallets must also be specified. Patterns that allow good circulation of gas to all parts of the load, designed with free space and "chimneys," are best from a sterilization standpoint but may conflict with commercial considerations. Sterility assurance, cycle duration, sterilizer capacity, and throughput rates are inextricably linked to validated loading patterns for ethylene oxide sterilization. A further factor involved in determining loading patterns is the rigors of ethylene oxide sterilization, which can affect the strength of corrugated cardboard. Partial or total collapse of a stacked pallet may involve some compromise of sterility. The use of "dividers" to give greater structural support to stacked pallets may impede gas penetration. All of these factors can only be addressed empirically; any significant change to a successful loading pattern must be validated thoroughly.

If more than one product is to be sterilized at the same time in the same sterilizer, process validation should be completed for each combination. The lot size in many manufacturing operations is "tailored" to sterilizer capacity, and in such instances it should not be difficult to avoid mixed loads. This may be more difficult for contract sterilization operations. Ethylene oxide sterilization contracts should address the validation of mixed loads or prohibit them. Both routes have cost implications.

The types of pallets should be specified—wood, aluminum, or some other material. Ethylene oxide is not absorbed by metal pallets, but the same cannot be said for wood. Wood is commonly used but difficult to control. Hard woods may absorb differently from soft woods, and some pallets may be water saturated, while others may be quite dry. Some of the unexpected and unpredictable sterilization failures seen in ethylene oxide sterilization may be associated with use of wood pallets. Once validated, change from one type of material to another should not be permitted.

2. *Equipment Specification*: Any change in process equipment or any introduction of new process equipment should be considered for validation. Biological validation may not always be necessary if there is sufficient physical or chemical evidence to demonstrate equivalence. All equipment should be identified; specifications, drawings, and instruction and maintenance manuals should be obtained and referenced in validation documentation. No list of equipment requiring validation can profess to be comprehensive. All functional equipment should be subject to scheduled inspection and preventative maintenance programs. All measuring devices must be calibrated and scheduled for regular recalibration.

a. External Preconditioning Chambers. External preconditioning chambers are not required to be as elaborate as sterilizers. This may in some cases lead to the belief that they are of only minor significance to the assurance of sterility. This is not correct. Due care and attention must be given to the design and specification of external preconditioning chambers.

They may be built to hold more than one sterilizer load, but if all loads are not to be removed at the same time some alarm or device should control the length of time that access doors are left open. This should be minimal. Preconditioning chambers should be of sufficient size to allow free circulation of air and moisture to all parts of the loads. The criteria for temperature and humidity specified for preconditioning rooms should be identical or very close to those obtaining in the sterilizer; in practice that means something close to those found in a sauna but less pleasant. The finish of preconditioning rooms should be robust enough to tolerate these conditions. Forced air circulation is necessary to the attainment of uniform conditions; fans should be equipped with alarms to indicate any failure.

Temperature and humidity in the preconditioning chamber should be specified and continuously monitored and recorded. These criteria should be related to the temperature and humidity obtained within the load. The object of preconditioning is to equilibrate the load to the conditions of the sterilizer; sufficient holding time in the preconditioning chamber should be specified to allow this to happen.

A maximum time limit between removal of a load from the preconditioning chamber and the commencement of sterilization should be specified. This may be particularly important in low-humidity locations.

b. Sterilizers and Ancillary Equipment. Allowing for all the normal criteria that apply to pressure vessels used for sterilization, the most important considerations to be specified for ethylene oxide sterilizers are the devices that contribute to the reproducibility and uniformity of control. Forced circulation may be necessary, and any such devices, as in the case of preconditioning chambers, should be specified to have alarms to indicate failure.

Gas concentration must be specified and demonstrated to be achieved. There are three methods for control and monitoring available. There are direct methods involving infrared analysis or gas chromatography. However, indirect methods are more robust and for that reason ought to be specified either on their own or alongside direct methods. Use of a sensitive, vulnerable, direct method of gas concentation without indirect backup in large-scale ethylene oxide sterilizers is usually seen to be an unacceptable commercial risk.

The most commonly used indirect method is by measurement of differential pressure within the sterilizer by means of pressure recorders. This method is permissible and valid only when using gas sources that are certified by the supplier, as it depends totally upon the differential pressure arising from ethylene oxide and not from some other gas. The gas concentration can be related to pressure and temperature through the formula

$$c = \frac{K \times MW \times P}{T}$$

where c = gas concentration (mg/L); MW = the molecular weight of the gas (MW of ethylene oxide = 44); K = a constant, 732.2; P = the increase in pressure in inches of Hg; and T = temperature in °Rankeine (460 + °F).

The second indirect method is by measurement of the weight of ethylene oxide delivered from the feed containers to the sterilizer. This method assumes no leakage, liquefaction, or polymerization of ethylene oxide in the gas lines connecting the gas source to the sterilizer. It is recommended that the two indirect methods be used in conjunction with each other. The weight loss method ensures that the increase in pressure is in fact due to gas from the ethylene oxide feed container and not from diluent gas or some other source; whereas the pressure method provides an ongoing index of gas concentration during the exposure period. Gas makeups should be automated and specified to be drawn from the ethylene oxide feed tanks, not from the diluent gas. Gas makeup may be controlled by pressure switches or by pressure transducers connected to solenoid valves controlling gas flow.

Direct methods of measuring gas concentration include gas chromatography and infrared spectroscopy. Both methods are dependent upon small samples, and the problems of drawing these samples should not be underestimated. The location of multiple sample ports should be such that a representative sample of a hopefully homogeneous gas mixture is obtainable. With most sterilizers operating at positive pressures, it is not usually necessary to have any special means of withdrawing the gas, but it is essential to have sample lines heated and insulated to avoid condensation of gas and water between the sterilizer and the analytical instrument.

Both gas chromatography and infrared analysis are dependent upon the instrumentation being calibrated against certified ethylene oxide supplies. Gas chromatography results are obtained as mol %, values which must then be converted to specifications defined in mg/L. Infrared results are directly correlated to mg/L.

Chamber temperature should be controllable and monitored throughout all cycles. The temperature obtained in a load is a function of the initial product temperature and its specific heat, the amount of steam injected, and the effectiveness of the insulation or the jacket at preventing heat loss. Temperature during the exposure phase of ethylene oxide sterilization cycles is not controlled by steam injection into the chamber as occurs in thermal sterilization. Loss of temperature may be compensated for by steam injection into the jacket. The control probe is usually located within the chamber rather than within the jacket, and control of temperature is a good deal less fine than in steam sterilizers because of the slower response through the jacket. Ethylene oxide sterilizers should be equipped with both jacket and chamber temperature indicators, and with chamber temperature recorders. Sterilizers should be specified with access ports to allow chamber and load temperature profiles to be obtained for the purposes of process validation.

Measurement of the humidity in the chamber and in the load has the least satisfactory technology of all the critical parameters of ethylene oxide sterilization. Direct measurement with gas chromatography or infrared analysis may not be reliable in the presence of ethylene oxide. Specification of the pressure increase obtained from steam injection is normally thought to be a satisfactory means of controlling humidity, but it does not offer a monitoring option.

The time of exposure may be manually or automatically controlled. Other time factors must also be specified and alarmed because they may affect sterility assurance in an unpredictable fashion or they may be indicative of other process problems. These time factors include the rate of evacuation at the beginning and at the end of the cycle, and the rate of increase of pressure as a result of gas injection.

For air ingress at the end of the cycle, ethylene oxide sterilizers should be equipped with sterilizing filters. Although the primary packaging material ought to have been chosen to be a barrier to microbial ingress, there remains the possibility that the significant pressure differentials and air flow rates that are obtained at the end of sterilization may be beyond validated tolerances.

The condition of the gas vaporizer is a further important consideration to ethylene oxide sterilization. All cylinder supplies of ethylene oxide present the gas in liquid form under pressure, which must then be vaporized before admission to the sterilizer. Inadequate temperatures in vaporizers may lead to the introduction of liquid ethylene oxide into the sterilizer. This is undesirable because it will not fulfill its purpose and because of staining and damage to product and packaging. Overly high temperatures may lead to degradation of the ethylene oxide with resultant polymer buildup restricting gas flow in the feed lines.

3. Process Validation (Physical): The equipment and the proposed preconditioning and operating cycles must be carefully specified in detail and with tight tolerances before starting process validation studies.

Multiprobe temperature and humidity distribution profiles should be obtained for empty preconditioning chambers, and temperature penetration profiles should be obtained with probes located within loads. The purpose of these studies is to demonstrate that the load is being uniformly equilibrated to the temperature (and by inference to the humidity) of the sterilizer within the proposed preconditioning time frame. Any serious lack of uniformity detected during validation studies should be investigated and corrected (even if only by extending the time of the preconditioning cycle).

It is normal practice to run large preconditioning chambers under operational conditions at all times irrespective of whether they are in use or not. If it is intended to use them on an ad hoc basis, validation studies should also cover the time taken for the chamber and the load to attain specified operating conditions.

The sterilizer and its associated pipework should be tested to ensure that it is adequate to maintain the positive pressures and vacuum pressures proposed in the cycle specification. The main thrust of physical validation is through temperature profiles.

Replicate temperature distribution profiles (from 3 to 24 sensors per cycle according to the size of the sterilizer) should be obtained for empty sterilizers operated to the proposed cycle specification. All parameters should be within their specified tolerances throughout validation cycles. For economic reasons an inert gas may be substituted for ethylene oxide in these studies. The *AAMI Guideline for Industrial Ethylene Oxide Sterilization of Medical Devices* [6] allows a variation of ± 3°C about the nominal specified temperature; sterilizer manufacturers [7] claim ± 2°C to be possible, this being a function of the types of controller used and of jacket design. At least one empty chamber temperature distribution profile should be run using ethylene oxide to discern whether there are any significant changes when the sterilant is being injected. Problems with vaporizers may be revealed by this means.

Empty chamber studies are sterilizer specific. Further process validation work is product specific (load specific) and may be done with dummy product if required. If this option is exercised, care must be taken to ensure that dummy loads are truly representative of genuine product. Scrap product is ideal for this purpose but may not be readily available for high cost products (e.g., cardiac pacemakers). If good product is used in validation, it should not be released as sterile until the validation program has been completed and signed off as satisfactory.

Load configurations and packaging materials have a significant effect on the rate of heat transfer into the product. Since it is microorganisms within the product that are to be inactivated, it is to the product that the critical process conditions must be delivered. Multiprobe temperature penetration profiles over replicate cycles are necessary. A wider tolerance of ± 5°C can be expected [6] due to slower response times. Cold spots (if any) should be identified and corrected, or specifically examined in the biological phase of process validation.

4. Process Validation (Biological): Biological validation is the most critical element of process validation of ethylene oxide sterilization. It is the only method of integrating the interaction of gas concentration, humidity, temperature, time, sterilizer effects, load effects, etc. It must demonstrate that the SAL being obtained is no worse than 10^{-6}, and it must demonstrate uniformity of treatment and it must provide the basis for routine monitoring. It is the only guarantee that the specifications for product and for process achieve sterility. Some preliminary work done in laboratory-scale sterilizers may provide favor-

able indications, but in the end trials must be done with actual product in a production-scale sterilizer.

The microorganisms used for biological validation of ethylene oxide sterilization are the spores of *Bacillus subtilis* var *niger (Bacillus globigii)*. These
spores are quite resistant to ethylene oxide though not the most resistant known.
They are indicator organisms. The spores are stable over time and ranges of
storage temperatures, and they are easily recognizable in culture because their
growth has an orange pellicle. However, exactly what constitutes a satisfactory
biological monitor using these spores and what constitutes an unsatisfactory
biological monitor continues to be a subject of debate.

The topic of biological validation of ethylene oxide sterilization processes
can be subdivided under two headings, microbiological monitor systems and
process challenge systems.

a. Microbiological Monitor Systems. The most contentious issue surrounding the use of biological monitors for validation and routine control of
ethylene oxide sterilization is that criteria for standardization have never been
described sufficiently well for there to have been international acceptance in the
manner that physical and chemical standards have been accepted. Standardization has been attempted by various organizations, for instance the USP and the
U.K. Department of Health.

All attempts at standardization have agreed that certain general characteristics of biological monitors should be specified; these are to use a recognized
strain of microorganism, to specify the number of microorganisms per monitor,
to specify a *D*-value, and to specify an expiry date.

Only the first of these characteristics (use of spores of *B. subtilis* var *niger*
ATCC 9372 or NCTC 10073) is without some form of complication with regard
to ethylene oxide monitors.

Even the standardization of numbers of spores per monitor is not straightforward. The numbers of spores recovered from monitors is not likely to
correspond to the numbers inoculated. The choice of carrier, the method of
loading the spores onto the carrier, and the methods of spore removal and
recovery may influence differences from the specified number. For instance,
because of the fibrous nature of papers, it is easier to remove spores from
aluminum carriers than from paper carriers. This does not necessarily mean that
aluminum carriers are better than paper carriers for the purposes of monitoring
sterilization cycles. Other variables related to adherence include "wettability"
and the speed and manner in which a spore suspension spreads across the
surfaces of a carrier, perhaps spreading evenly, perhaps forming clumps. This
makes it difficult to translate a specified number of spores per carrier into a
process for preparing consistent biological monitors.

Commercially available spore strips are usually intended to have 10^6
viable recoverable spores per strip. They may be loaded onto carriers by indi-

vidual inoculation or by running a carrier strip through a bath of spore suspension at a controlled rate.

The response of particular microorganisms to particular sterilization processes is usually improved through the D-value. However, the D-value of spores used to monitor ethylene oxide sterilization processes is of less relevance to practical sterilization than D-values of microorganisms versus other sterilization processes. If biological monitors were to be used in conjunction with gamma radiation sterilization (noting that this is not necessary), the D_{10}-value versus the single parameter of absorbed dose would be directly relatable across all cobalt-60 gamma irradiators. D_T values for thermal sterilization processes are transferrable from one autoclave, oven, or tunnel to another. With ethylene oxide this is not the case; the D-value of a spore population is relevant only to the conditions of gas concentration, temperature, humidity, time of exposure, and gassing up and degassing times for which it was determined.

Attempts have been made to standardize at least the conditions in which D-values may be determined, AAMI [8] have specified a sterilizing vessel, termed a biological indicator evaluator resistometer (BIER vessel), which allows rapid attainment and termination of exposure conditions in a precise and accurate manner.

The time to reach target gas concentration must be less than 60 s, and gas concentration is specified as 600 mg/L ± 30 mg/L at 54°C ± 1°C and 50 to 70% RH. The time to exhaust a BIER vessel must be less than 60 s and accurate to ± 10 s. It would be an unusual production sterilizer that could conform to these criteria.

In addition to these fundamental problems of translating ethylene oxide D-values from one situation to another, the D-value obtained even in the best-controlled BIER vessel may be affected quite significantly by the methods used to prepare the monitors and the methods used to determine resistance.

Most significantly, biological monitors prepared at different levels of dryness do not respond in the same manner to ethylene oxide inactivation.

In other words, the D-value is a function of the previous history of the monitor as well as of the sterilizer in which it was determined. The composition of the fluid from which the spores were dried may also influence D-values by coating the spores with a layer of material through which moisture or ethylene oxide may have restricted permeability. This also gives importance to the conditions in which the spores were grown (complex or defined media) and washed. Graham [10] quotes D-values of 2.4 min and 3.5 min for the same strain of $B.$ subtilis var niger grown in different liquid media and exposed to ethylene oxide under identical conditions.

Finally, the requirement to specify an expiry date implies that something is going to deteriorate or change over time. The most obvious characteristics are numbers of spores per monitor (do the spores die over time? do they lose adherence to the carrier over time?) and D-values. Stability over time can only be determined empirically; again, it is likely to be a function of the biological monitor itself and of the method of preparation of the biological monitor.

b. Process Challenge Systems. Broadly there are three methods by which microbiological monitor organisms may be presented as process challenges. These are

(a) Inoculated carriers. These are generally in the form of spore strips; strips of paper or aluminum inoculated with spores of *B. subtilis* var *niger*. Commercially available spore strips are usually individually packed in glassine envelopes.

(b) Self-contained biological monitors. These are sophisticated variants of inoculated carriers in which the recovery medium is an integral part of the monitor. For ethylene oxide the spores are mounted on a carrier that is in one compartment of a two-compartment unit. In the other compartment is the recovery medium. After exposure, the seal between the two compartments is broken open and the surviving spores (if any) are incubated in the medium.

(c) Inoculated products. A very small proportion of the total number of biological monitors used to challenge ethylene oxide sterilization processes will be actual product samples carrying an inoculum of spores. Theoretically this is the most valuable indicator of sterility assurance. In most cases it loses out to practicality. Many medical products are too bulky to incubate *in situ*, and even if this were overcome the amount of medium and incubator space required to cater for large numbers of biological monitors of this type might soon become prohibitive. Removal of spores from the inoculated device into some other carrier for incubation introduces a further variable and increases the complexity of laboratory manipulations.

Of the three types of carrier, the spore strip is the most commonly used. Once this choice is made there are several other essential decisions.

The first of these is where to place the microbiological monitor in the product. The ruling is that it should be placed in the location most difficult to sterilize. To some extent this is a reflection of professional judgement. It is a curious anomaly that most ethylene oxide sterilizers of hypodermic products judge the most difficult position within the product to be between the two "lands" or "ribs" of the plunger tip because this is an enclosed cavity. However, at the same time, it is also the location where ethylene oxide is most likely to persist longest because of its preferential absorption into rubber. The location most difficult to sterilize may not be amenable to placement of biological monitors. In these circumstances it is usually recommended to use some other product or device packed in a similar or identical manner to simulate the actual product.

The number of spores per strip and the number of strips per load should for validation purposes be related in some way to the bioburden of the product. What type of relationship this should be is less obvious. There are two broad approaches to this; the first is to relate the microbiological challenge on each spore strip to the average bioburden on individual products and the required level of sterility assurance (SAL); the second is to relate the total microbiological challenge in the sterilizer load to the total bioburden within the sterilizer.

Both approaches require some estimation of product bioburden. It is not advisable for ethylene oxide sterilization processes to be validated without at least some estimates of numbers of product contaminants. This is irrespective of whether cycle development is by the so-called overkill or the so-called bioburden method (see below).

If the number of spores per load is to be related to the total bioburden of the load, the average bioburden per item must be multiplied by the number of items in the load to give an estimate of the total bioburden in the load. The number of spore strips to be used in validation may be calculated by dividing this number by the number of spores per biological monitor thus

$$\text{Number of spore strips per load} = N_0 \times \frac{m}{C}$$

where N_0 = the average number of contaminants per item prior to sterilization, m = the number of items per load, and C = the number of spores per biological monitor.

If the number of spores per spore strip and the number of spores per validation load is to be related to the individual product item and a sterility assurance level of 10^{-6}, it is first necessary to know the average number of contaminants per product item. In the interests of conservatism this number may be rounded up or supplemented by a safety factor. The target is to use as many spore strips as is necessary to provide assurance that this bioburden is being inactivated to an SAL of 10^{-6}. This can be calculated from

$$\text{Number of spores per load} = N_0 + \frac{1}{\text{SAL}}$$

where N_0 = the average number of contaminants per item prior to sterilization and SAL = the required sterility assurance level.

The number of spore strips per load can be obtained by dividing this figure by the number of spores per strip.

Given that these methods can provide a means of deciding how many biological monitors should be used for validation purposes, there are two approaches to cycle validation. These have been termed overkill and bioburden.

An overkill cycle is quite simply one that inactivates the microbiological challenge plus an additional safety factor. As a rule of thumb, the shortest exposure time obtained in validation runs that will consistently inactivate all of the microbiological challenge organisms should be doubled to specify an adequate overkill cycle.

Bioburden cycles normally require resistance data as well as estimates of numbers of microbial contaminants. In this respect AAMI are using the term bioburden in its broadest sense, almost as a synonym for microflora.

Resistance work cannot be done in large-scale production sterilizers, because the gassing and degassing times are too long. These must be done in laboratory-scale equipment or BIER vessels. They should be done preferably for microorganisms actually isolated from the product and with microbiological monitors. A comparison should be made of the resistance (D-values) of both types of microorganism in simple situations (say on strips held in glass petri dishes) and in product items or simulated product items. The cycle should be chosen on the basis of the determined resistance of the bioburden being sufficiently treated within the specified parameters to provide a 10^{-6} SAL. Final proof of this must be obtained with microbiological monitors in the production sterilizer. As an example, assuming that the average bioburden per item is equal to n microorganisms of D-value D_b, the exposure time for a 10^{-6} SAL may be calculated from

$$\text{Exposure time} = D_b \cdot (\log n + 6)$$

The number of spores per biological monitor required to be inactivated to verify that this cycle is effective can then be calculated from

$$\text{Log number of spores per monitor} = D_b \cdot \frac{(\log n + 6)}{D_m}$$

where D_m = D-value of *Bacillus subtilis* var *niger*.

For validation purposes, microbiological monitors are intended not only to provide an index of achievement of SAL, but also to provide (among other things) some index of process uniformity. They must therefore be placed throughout the load in pallet positions close to and far from the entry ports for gas and steam, near the surfaces and deep within stacked pallets. Microbiological monitors should be placed alongside temperature sensors during validation, but it should be noted that the sensors may introduce a route for easier access of gas than might occur in their absence. The choice of locations for biological monitors is in the long run arbitrary.

B. Routine Control of Ethylene Oxide Sterilization

The emphasis for routine control of irradiation sterilization and thermal sterilization has been toward tight control of the physical parameters that lead to microbial inactivation rather than toward control through biological testing. At one time there would have been an emphasis on biological methods for controlling these other sterilization processes, but as the scientific basis of these processes has become better known, and their technology has become better controlled, biological monitoring has diminished in importance. This is not yet the case with ethylene oxide sterilization. Both biological and physical methods of monitoring are absolutely necessary to provide reasonable assurance of sterility.

The first requirement of a routine monitoring program for ethylene oxide sterilization is specification of the critical parameters. Any excursion beyond the specified tolerances for any one of these critical parameters must stimulate rejection or resterilization irrespective of whether biological monitoring criteria are met. This acknowledges the fallibility of biological monitoring methods and the limitations on the numbers of biological monitors that may be used practically. The instrumentation used to monitor these characteristics must be independent of the instrumentation used for control.

Other excursions beyond less critical specifications and tolerances should be noted as a matter of routine in the event of these providing an early warning of some progressive deterioration or loss of control that may in the long run impact upon sterility or safety, for instance wear and tear on vacuum pumps.

The second critical requirement for routine monitoring is a biological monitoring system. Biological monitors should be placed in the product load, retrieved promptly after sterilization finishes, be left for a controlled period to lose any residues or traces of ethylene oxide, and then cultivated in appropriate recovery media.

Fewer biological monitors are needed for routine monitoring than would be used for validation. There should be some concentration on cold spots (if any), but at the same time there should be some attempt at random or representative covering of all parts of the sterilizer and of the load. The history and reproducibility of particular ethylene oxide sterilization technologies may influence the confidence that can be placed on a particular process. Precise and reproducible technology does not merit as much biological monitoring as less reliable equipment. A sound sterilization history of a particular sterilizer coupled with a particular cycle and a particular product does not require as much biological monitoring as a new sterilizer, new product, or new cycle. How many biological monitors is a matter of professional judgement.

Most biological monitoring is done on a quantal response (growth/no growth) basis, and if any one biological monitor shows growth the load should be rejected or resterilized. Once again this decision should be made independently and irrespective of whether physical process specifications have been met. This acknowledges the empiricism of the ethylene oxide sterilization process. With so many variables it can be quite possible to fail to achieve sterilizing conditions at some point or points locally in the load. If there is biological evidence of this having happened the decision can only be the conservative one.

Spores of *B. subtilis* var *niger* form an orange pellicle in simple standard recovery media, so failure is easy to recognize and simple to distinguish from incidental contamination. Laboratories with high incidences of incidental contamination should seriously review their procedures for recovering biological monitors from the sterilizer and from the product. They should also review their aseptic techniques. This emphasis acknowledges that microorganisms compete for nutrients such that faster growing contaminants may obscure survival of the biological monitor.

One of the major commercial difficulties with biological monitoring is the incubation of the biological monitors. Various sources may recommend 7, 10, or 14 days. With reliable technology and a satisfactory sterilization history it is quite reasonable to divorce the incubation of biological monitors from the shipment of product from the sterilization site, as long as the product is not actually put into use and is accountable and retrievable in the event of a subsequent biological failure. This is not parametric release, but a commercial risk, and it should be exercised with considerable care and only when processes subsequent to sterilization but concurrent with incubation, e.g., degassing, packing, and labelling in shippers, transportation, and warehousing, operate over a time scale that ensures that nonsterile product is unlikely to reach the final user before completion of incubation.

In addition to the use of biological monitors it is also advisable with ethylene oxide sterilization processes to include a routine batch-by-batch pharmacopoeial sterility test. Its statistical limitations remain as a barrier to its value for confirming sterility. However, it should not be discounted as a further means of investigating the possibility of failure to achieve sterility (i.e., as a test for nonsterility) in a poorly predictable situation.

V. HEALTH AND SAFETY

Ethylene oxide damages biological systems. Its effects are not peculiar to microorganisms, but apply to all biological systems. Ethylene oxide and its by-products are toxic, mutagenic, and carcinogenic to animals and humans. Ideally ethylene oxide residues should not be present on medical products. In practice there are technologies available to ensure that the use of ethylene oxide need not result in an unacceptably high risk to human health.

Acute effects of ethylene oxide and its by-product ethylene chlorhydrin (CH_2ClCH_2OH), formed by reaction with chloride ions, include symptoms of nausea, dizziness, and signs of mental disturbance. Ethylene chlorhydrin may also cause kidney and liver degeneration. The most serious effects of both substances may lead to cancer. Exposure to ethylene oxide induces irreversible chromosomal aberrations (sister chromatid exchange) and other precancerous changes in the peripheral lymphocytes.

There are two broad groups at risk. The first of these comprises ethylene oxide sterilization workers who are subject to exposure by inhalation and perhaps to skin contact with liquid ethylene oxide while changing gas cylinders. The second group comprises the recipients of ethylene oxide sterilized products, including patients who may be receiving treatment and medical or nursing staff who must come into regular and frequent contact with ethylene oxide sterilized products.

The group at highest risk are sterilization workers, patients on hemodyalysis equipment, and persistent users of hypodermic equipment (e.g., diabetics using insulin syringes) and habitual users of ethylene oxide sterilized gloves. There is a middle risk category of patients on intravenous therapy using ethylene oxide sterilized infusion sets over a comparatively short period of time. In numbers this is the largest group. The lowest risk is to patients who receive one time implants (e.g., cardiac pacemakers), one single dose of ethylene oxide absorbed completely.

The most stringent attitudes to worker protection have been those of the Occupational Safety and Health Administration in the U.S.A. There are three limit standards to be considered. The permissible exposure limit (PEL) is a measure of good industrial hygiene practice expressed as an 8-h time weighted average (TWA8). The PEL set by OSHA is 1 ppm TWA8 measured in a manner representative of the employees' breathing zone. Personnel are subject to medical surveillance; areas where greater ethylene oxide exposure may be expected must be identified, respiratory protection must be provided for particular tasks, and risks should be identified through appropriate signs and labels. If an action limit of 0.5 ppm TWA8 is being consistently achieved, then the frequency of medical surveillance and monitoring may be reduced. The third limit is an excursion limit (EL) not to be exceeded over a 15-min period. This has been set at 5 ppm.

In Europe PELs for ethylene oxide range from 1 ppm TWA8 in Belgium and Denmark through 5 ppm TWA8 in the U.K. and France up to 50 ppm TWA8 in the Netherlands. France has a 15-min EL of 10 ppm.

Surrounding these limits are a series of complications. In general PELs can be attained by use of segregated areas for ethylene oxide sterilization and ethylene oxide storage. Ventilation is of utmost importance, and, since ethylene oxide is heavier than air, low-level exhaust systems are to be preferred. Other engineering measures may include interlocks and remote control consoles. Short-term excursion limits (ELs) may necessitate positive pressure self-contained respiratory protection to be used for particular tasks, for instance unloading sterilizers and changing gas cylinders. Personal protection should not, however, be considered until it can be shown conclusively that ELs cannot be achieved by engineering controls or changed workplace practices.

Ethylene oxide residues remaining on products present a more complicated picture. Limits should properly be based on risk assessment. Satisfactory risk assessment involves an analysis of a multitude of complex factors concerning particular medical products, their frequency of usage, and the characteristics of the recipients. Some still unfinalized residue limits provided by the FDA in 1978 provide a guideline to appropriate targets. These range from 5 to 250 ppm by weight of device depending on the type of device [11]. By and large these recommendations follow the risk categories described previously. There is some conjecture over ppm by weight of device being the most appropriate measure to define limits. In many cases surface area in contact with the recipient's tissue or in contact with fluids being infused may be argued to be more appropriate.

Methods of extraction and analysis have been published by the Association for the Advancement of Medical Instrumentation [12]. Water or other aqueous systems are most commonly used for extraction. Two extraction methods are recommended, exhaustive extraction and simulated use. In fact both methods, if used correctly, represent simulated use. Exhaustive extraction is recommended for devices such as implants, which by merit of their prolonged contact with tissue over time can be expected to transfer all of their residual ethylene oxide to the recipient. Simulated use extraction of a less exhaustive nature might include fluid path extraction over a simulated maximum hold period for infusion sets and hypodermic syringes. Analysis is by gas chromatography.

There are four ways in which ethylene oxide may be retained in products at the end of sterilization cycles. These are as gaseous ethylene oxide, as ethylene oxide dissolved in water, as ethylene oxide within but not attached to the product or packaging material, and as molecularly adsorbed or absorbed ethylene oxide [13]. The total amount of residual ethylene oxide and the balance among the four forms of residue at the end of sterilization are functions of the sterilization process conditions, the composition of the product, the size of the product, the packaging materials, and the packing density. Dissipation of residues after sterilization is a function of the product- and packaging-related factors listed above plus the conditions in which the product is being held (aeration).

The amount of residual ethylene oxide in a product can be significantly influenced by sterilization process conditions. Gas concentrations and exposure times within the exposure period of the cycle should be sufficient to achieve sterility, but their effects on residues should be considered before prolonging them unnecessarily. Importantly, free gaseous ethylene oxide is easiest to remove from product loads, and this is best addressed by postexposure evacuation and aeration. Multiple evacuations and forced circulation aeration at temperatures around 30°C have been found to be effective. The effects of increased temperatures extend beyond the removal of the free gas to the removal of other forms of bound ethylene oxide.

After removal of the load from the sterilizer, further dissipation of residues is a function of time, temperature, and ventilation. Generally, the rate of ethylene oxide dissipation doubles for every 10°C rise in temperature (the Q_{10} is equal to 2), and ventilation should be sufficient to maintain a concentration gradient between the ethylene oxide in the product and the ethylene oxide in the atmosphere. Movement of ethylene oxide from the product into the atmosphere is governed by Fick's laws of diffusion. Given that there are technological and commercial restrictions on the conditions in which ethylene oxide sterilized products can be held after sterilization and before release to the market, serious consideration should be given to the ways in which product and packaging composition and design can affect the dissipation of ethylene oxide.

It is paradoxical that the abilities of ethylene oxide to penetrate materials that make it an effective sterilant are the same abilities that create residues. Polymeric materials are very permeable to ethylene oxide. Permeability is affected by the solubility of the gas in the polymer and the diffusivity of the polymer to ethylene oxide. Ethylene oxide is less soluble in polyethylene and polyesters (around 10,000 ppm) than in say cellulosics or PVC (around 30,000 to 40,000 ppm according to the level of plasticizers present in the formulation); soft plastics and natural rubbers have higher diffusion coefficients for ethylene oxide than harder polymers such as acrylics and styrenes [14]. Polymers with high diffusion coefficients will reach saturation solubility quicker than those with lower diffusion coefficients. A polymer that takes up residues only slowly will release them only slowly. Since devices may often be manufactured with several different types of polymeric material, it is difficult to predict or quantify overall residue levels and practical rates of dissipation. A component such as the rubber plunger tip may as a result of its high diffusivity and thickness amount for most of the residues in a hypodermic syringe, although it is in itself only a minor component.

Much of what has been said about the movement of ethylene oxide in and out of products also applies to packaging materials. Primary packaging materials are only very rarely of a significant thickness, and should be chosen to allow rapid penetration of ethylene oxide to the product during the exposure period of the sterilization cycle. They should therefore present an insignificant barrier to the dissipation of residues. Molecules released from the product dissolve in the permeable primary packaging materials on the side with the higher concentration and diffuse in the direction of the concentration gradient toward the side with the lower concentration of ethylene oxide. The residues desorb to the atmosphere on the side of lower concentration.

In the long run, corrugated cardboard boxes and wooden pallets may allow residues to hang around the load and the product longer than necessary. Loads should not be left to aerate in conditions where ventilation may be restricted by too great packing densities or where some pallets may occlude air movement around others.

REFERENCES

1. Dadd, A. H., and Daley, G. M. (1980). Resistance of microorganisms to inactivation by gaseous ethylene oxide. *Journal of Applied Bacteriology* **49**: 89 101.
2. Ernst, R. R. (1973). Ethylene oxide gaseous sterilization for industrial applications. In *Industrial Sterilization* (G. Briggs Phillips and W. S. Miller, eds.). Durham, N.C.: Duke University Press.
3. Ernst, R. R., and Doyle, J. E. (1968). Sterilization with gaseous ethylene oxide: A review of chemical and physical factors. *Biotechnology and Bioengineering* **10**: 1–31.
4. Kaye, S., and Phillips, C. R. (1949). The sterilizing action of ethylene oxide IV. The effect of moisture. *American Journal of Hygiene* **50**: 296–306.
5. Dadd, A. H., and Daley, G. M. (1982). Role of the coat in resistance of bacterial spores to inactivation by ethylene oxide. *Journal of Applied Bacteriology* **53**: 109–116.
6. Association for the Advancement of Medical Instrumentation (1981). *Guideline for Industrial Ethylene Oxide Sterilization of Medical Devices*. Arlington, Va.: AAMI.
7. Skocypec, R. (1984). Installation and equipment performance qualification of gas sterilizers. In *Sterilization Validation of Medical Devices and Surgical Products*. EUCOMED International Conference, May 16-17, 1984.
8. Association for the Advancement of Medical Instrumentation (1982). *Standard for Biological Indicator Evaluator Resistometer (BIER) Ethylene Oxide Vessels*. Arlington, Va.: AAMI.
9. Pattinson, D. H. (1986). Rehumidification of biological indicators. In *Proceedings of EUCOMED Workshop on Biological Monitoring of Sterilization*. Kerkrade, Netherlands, April 21-23, 1986.
10. Graham, G. (1986). Production of spores and preparation of spore suspensions and monitors. In *Proceedings of EUCOMED Workshop on Biological Monitoring of Sterilization*. Kerkrade, Netherlands, April 21-23, 1986.
11. Rodricks, J. V., and Brown, S. L. (1991). Ethylene oxide residues: Toxicity, risk assessment, and standards. In *Sterilization of Medical Products Volume V* (R. F. Morrissy and Y. Prokopenko, eds.). Morin Heights, Canada: Polyscience Publications.
12. Association for the Advancement of Medical Instrumentation (1986). *Recommended Practice for Determining Residual Ethylene Oxide in Medical Devices*. Arlington, Va.: AAMI.
13. Lyon, M. (1988). Comparison of sterilization cycles for EtO residuals. *Medical Device and Diagnostic Industry* **10**: 20–24.
14. Manning, C. R. (1989). Controlling EtO residues from the manufacture of medical products. *Medical Device and Diagnostic Industry* **11**: 136–144.

Sterilization by Filtration

Microbial inactivation is not the only way of achieving sterility. A major alternative to killing microorganisms contaminating medical and pharmaceutical products is to remove them from the products. Filtration is one means of doing this for fluids.

Filtration does not rely on chemical reaction to inactivate microorganisms; it is therefore suitable for heat-labile and radiation-sensitive fluids. Filtration should leave no traces nor leach chemical contaminants into the product. As a continuous or semicontinuous process it is suitable for sterilization of volumes of fluids that might be prohibitively large for other methods of batch sterilization.

Modern methods of filtration can be as reliable a mechanism of sterilization as methods relying on biochemical inactivation of microorganisms. Filtration in its simplest sense of removal of particles from a fluid by passage of the fluid through a medium that has pores large enough to allow the fluid to pass but too small to allow the particles to pass (sieving) is only one component of a highly complex process.

I. MEMBRANE FILTRATION

Sterile filtration of liquids and gases is now virtually always done using membrane filters. The first U.S. patent for membrane filters was filed in 1922 and pertained to cellulose acetate membranes. A wide range of membrane filter media are now commercially available to suit various applications: cellulose esters, polyvinylidinefluoride, polytetrafluoroethylene (PTFE), and polyhexamethyleneadipamide (nylon 66), separately or as laminates with polyethylene, polypropylene, and polyester for more robust physical characteristics.

Membrane filters are thin, uniform porous sheets that in the older scientific literature were described to be acting as screens or sieves that trapped on their surfaces all particles larger in size than the pores in the membrane or larger than the interstices of the mesh of the membranes. This type of particle removal is absolute in the sense of it being independent of the filtration conditions. Sieving is not influenced by pressure differentials nor by the chemical or physical properties of the fluid unless these are sufficient to deform, damage, or otherwise alter the size of the pores. Particle entrapment by sieving alone is now known to be an excessively simplistic interpretation of what happens to particles during membrane filtration.

Physical sieving or surface retention of particles larger than the pores in the membrane is only one of several mechanisms of particle retention that may occur in membrane filters. In reality, membrane filters are also capable of retaining particles that are dimensionally smaller than their pores.

These other mechanisms of retaining particles within the depth of membranes may be mechanical or physicochemical. Mechanical means of entrapment apply equally to liquid and gas filtration; they include inertial impaction to the walls or surfaces of the pores and lodgement in crevices and "dead ends." Theoretical models and other illustrations of membrane filters often portray pores as being cylindrical in shape and as passing directly from the top surface of the membrane to the bottom surface by the shortest straightest route. In fact pores are rarely cylindrical, they do not have smooth walls, and their passage may be extremely convoluted even through very thin (typically 0.015 cm) depths of membrane. Physicochemical interactions with the filter medium can be very complex and differ according to the types of particles, the fluid in which they are suspended, and the dynamics of the filtration system. Electrostatic forces are of more importance in gas filtration than in liquid filtration. Adsorption of surfactants from liquid suspensions to both particles and pore surfaces may result in mutually repulsive ionic forces that encourage the passage of particles. On the other hand, retention of small particles may be favored in liquid suspensions through covalent bonding, and through attraction by van der Waals forces when zeta potentials of both particles and pore surfaces are low (usually less than 30 mV). Most particles carry a negative zeta potential in water; for this bonding mechanism to be operative in filtration it is necessary therefore for the membrane to have a positive zeta potential. Commercial membrane manufacturers offer charged media for specialized applications.

These other mechanisms may or may not occur in particular circumstances. All are reversible and all may reach saturation levels beyond which they are ineffective for particle retention. In the long run, reliance can only be placed on surface collection for absolute removal of particles from fluids. For sterilization purposes, the particles that must be retained by filters are microbiological ones. The FDA defines a sterilizing filter in terms of microbiological particle passage: "a sterilizing filter is one which, when challenged with the microorganism *Pseudomonas diminuta*, at a minimum concentration of 10^7 organisms per cm^2 of filter surface, will produce a sterile effluent" [1]. The possibility of mechanisms other than sieving contributing to microbial retention is acknowledged by the recognition that the number of particles in the challenge may be able to saturate the retention mechanisms of the filter. The FDA goes on, however, to relate satisfactory sterilizing membranes to a rated "porosity" of 0.22 μm or smaller, chosen because *Ps. diminuta* ATCC 19146 has an inherently small mean diameter of 0.3 μm. Regardless of whether membrane filtration's main mechanism of particle retention is sieving or some other means, pore size is clearly seen to be of significant importance to the choice of membranes to be used for sterilization.

A. Pore Size Rating

What is meant by the pore size ratings of commercially available membranes? Pore size ratings of commercially available membranes are not indices of maximum pore opening diameters obtained from direct microscopic measurement or by particle passage methods. Ratings are almost always determined by indirect means based on theoretical considerations and on nondestructive test technology.

Theoretical aspects of pore size rating have been addressed by Schroeder and DeLuca [2]. Wet membranes are impermeable to the flow of gas until a pressure is reached that is sufficiently high to dislodge the liquid from the pores (Fig. 1). The diameters of cylindrical pores can be calculated from this differen-

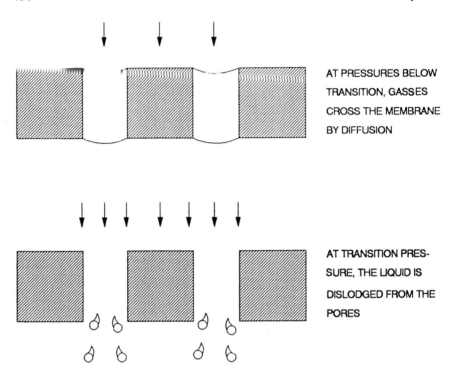

Fig. 1 Idealized displacement of liquid from pores.

tial pressure, termed the bubble point pressure, at which liquid is displaced from the pores of a wetted filter.

If membrane pores can be regarded as simple cylindrical capillaries, liquid will be held in the pores by surface tension forces described by the equation

$$d = 4y \cdot \frac{\cos \theta}{P}$$

where d = the diameter of the pore, y = the surface tension of the liquid filling the pore, P = the pressure required to overcome surface tension (the bubble point pressure), and θ = the contact angle between the liquid and the pore wall (if the contact angle is zero, $\cos \theta = 1$). This equation indicates an inverse relationship between pore diameter and bubble point; therefore if pressure is being increased gradually across a wetted membrane, the first signs of fluid displacement at lowest pressures will be from the largest pores. This provides the basis of an intrinsically conservative indirect method for determining theoretical pore size ratings.

Some examples of how theoretical pore diameters may be calculated from bubble point pressures are given in Annex 1.

The two functions y and θ relating to the wetting liquid indicate the specificity of the method to particular test conditions; for instance, if methanol were to be used as a wetting liquid, bubble points would be usually about one-third of those found with the same membrane if water were to be used as the wetting liquid.

For practical applications, an empirical nonideality factor K should be applied to correct for pores that do not have perfectly circular unbroken perimeters, thus

$$d = K \cdot 4y \cdot \frac{\cos \theta}{P}$$

Elliptical pores may be addressed theoretically. For ellipses with differing diameters it is the smallest diameter that is of significance in filtration because the sieving mechanism of the membrane can only be effective for particles larger than this dimension.

The surface tension forces that must be overcome to allow displacement of a liquid from a membrane are mainly a function of the size of the perimeter (the circumference) of the pore. The hydrostatic forces that promote displacement of the liquid are mainly a function of the area of the pore. At the bubble point, when these two sets of forces are in equilibrium, the smallest diameter d of an elliptical pore can be calculated from the equation

$$d = \frac{4y \cdot \cos \theta \ \sqrt{(1 + E^2)/2}}{EP}$$

where E = the ratio between the largest and smallest diameters of the ellipse.

This equation shows that, at any particular bubble point pressure, E is inversely proportional to d. Therefore the assumption of a pore being cylindrical ($E = 1$) will provide a higher estimate of d than any estimate obtained by correcting for the elliptical shape of the pore. To assume that the pore is cylindrical introduces an inaccuracy in the estimation of the pore's diameter; it is, however, a conservative inaccuracy.

Pore size ratings of commercially available membrane filters are usually based on bubble point pressure calculations. This is not to say that they are purely based on these theoretical considerations. Practical knowledge of the processes of manufacture of membranes, detailed knowledge of pore size distribution from electron microscope studies, correction factors to compensate for irregular pore peripheries, and other considerations are likely to be taken into account in determining ratings. Pore size ratings of say 0.22 μm from different manufacturers are not necessarily derived by the same method and should not therefore be assumed to be describing identical membranes.

Factually, one can expect to find membranes with specified pore size ratings to have a proportion of pores with larger diameters than the rating would suggest, yet quite capable of retaining microorganisms physically smaller than these pores. Electron microscope studies [3] of commercially available membranes that had pore size ratings of 0.22 μm and that had been shown to be capable of meeting the FDA's microbiological particle passage criterion revealed pores with diameters larger than 0.3 μm on their surfaces and throughout their depths. In summary, pore size rating cannot be correlated precisely to the size of the smallest microbiological particle that the membrane is capable of retaining.

B. Microbial Particle Passage

Pore size is clearly not the only factor influencing the retention of microorganisms on or in membrane filters. Other mechanisms in addition to sieving affect microbial retention. The FDA's microbial particle passage standard, that a sterilizing filter should be capable of retaining a challenge of at least 10^7 microorganisms of a particular type per cm^2, is an end-result criterion that does not by itself help to quantify measurable characteristics of membranes or membrane types that contribute to retention.

The design of microbial particle passage experiments is not without its microbiological complications (see Section III below), and since these tests are destructive of the material being tested they are not well suited to routine application. Microbial particle passage experimentation has, however, assisted in identifying some important factors involved in microbial retention. In principle, removal of bacteria from fluids by retention on or in membranes is simple to determine by challenging a filtration unit with a suspension of a known concentration of a specified microorganism, usually *Ps. diminuta*. An index of the filter's retention properties can be obtained by comparing the concentration of microorganisms in the challenge to the concentration of microorganisms recovered downstream.

In practice there is an upper limit to the number of microorganisms that can be used to challenge a membrane. This is determined by the open pore volume of the membrane and the pore size. The numbers of microorganisms trapped on the surface of a membrane affect the amount of open pore volume and therefore diminish flow (clogging). Particle size is also a factor, because pores are most effectively blocked by particles of about the same size as the pores. The most discriminating experimental conditions exist when all pores are being challenged by potential penetrants, i.e., when the challenge is sufficient to cover the membrane surface completely but below the clogging concentration. Scanning electron micrographs of this situation [4] show a double layer of cells of *Ps. diminuta* from a challenge concentration of 10^8 per cm^2 on the surface of 0.22 μm pore size rated membranes. When membranes become clogged, excessively high differential pressures are required to maintain a constant flow rate, and furthermore the proportion of the challenge population penetrating the membrane diminishes [3].

The performance characteristics of the membrane, flow rate and applied differential pressure, may also affect microbial particle passage experiments. The rate at which a liquid is able to pass through a membrane is defined by the equation

$$Q = C \cdot \frac{AP}{V}$$

where Q = flow rate, A = filtration area, P = differential pressure across the membrane, V = viscosity of the liquid, and C = resistance to flow by the membrane.

This equation indicates that at a constant differential pressure across the membrane, flow rate will decrease as the effective filtration area becomes clogged by particles. Experiments are normally performed, therefore, at constant differential pressure (usually in the range of 30–50 psig) but with a diminishing flow rate, or at a constant flow rate obtained by progressively increasing the differential pressure across the membrane.

For membranes with pore dimensions larger than those of *Ps. diminuta*, higher pressures pose a more severe challenge than lower pressures [4]. This suggests that entrapment of microorganisms in the tortuous passages of the pores is one of the main mechanisms of retention. Pall [5] describes particles as "stupid," blundering passively through pores, potentially deformable, squeezing themselves or being squeezed by pressure through narrower passages than they might otherwise traverse.

Pall [3] has also demonstrated that the proportion of the challenge population of *Ps. diminuta* passing through a membrane is approximately constant regardless of the initial size of the challenge. This implies that if a number of membranes of the same type were to be set up in series, each would remove the same proportion of its incoming challenge, and therefore that microbial retention by membrane filters is an exponential function similar to methods of sterilization involving microbial inactivation. The importance of this is in relation to the effect of membrane thickness on microbial retention; given two membranes with identical pore sizes (as a rating from bubble point pressure measurements, or as a direct measurement by some other means), the thicker of the two membranes provides greater assurance against microbial penetration. Membrane thickness may therefore be placed alongside pore size rating as an important index of the effectiveness of a sterilizing filter.

II. APPLICATIONS OF STERILIZING FILTRATION

There are two main occasions for the use of filtration in the sterilization of fluids. The first is when fluids are damaged or destroyed by exposure to other sterilization processes; the second is when the scale of sterilization is too large to be addressed through other sterilization processes.

Aseptic processing of liquid pharmaceutical formulations implies the use of sterile filtration. Filtration should not be the method of choice ahead of thermal sterilization, but it is not out of the question; some heat-stable pharmaceutical liquid products are currently being filter-sterilized and aseptically processed. Sterilizing membranes for this purpose should have a pore size rating no greater than 0.22 μm. It is normal to filter from a clean compounding area through an intact physical barrier into the aseptic filling room where the filling machines are located. There may be intermediate vessels, or filtration may be directly to the filling machine. It is good practice to mount a further sterilizing filter at or close to the point of fill.

Sterilizing filters for liquids are clearly a critical application of filtration. They are normally used for a limited period of time, discarded, and replaced with fresh filters for subsequent batches or campaigns of production. In other words, they are applied to relatively small-scale operations.

Sterile filtration of gases, particularly air, is frequently necessary in the pharmaceutical and medical products industries. Some gases may be heat sensitive, but filtration is used in the main because of the volumes of gas requiring sterilization. Gases may be used to "sparge" or "blanket" pharmaceutical formulations; compressed air may be used in their processing; air or oxygen may be required in large quantities for fermentation processes; water and other storage tanks may require their venting to be protected from contamination arising from airborne microbiological contamination. By and large, these filters remain in place far longer than liquid filters and indeed may be subject to repeated steam sterilization.

A. Construction of Sterilizing Filters

For all but the most unusual circumstances, there are two types of sterilizing filter available, disc and cartridge filters. With disc filters, the necessary surface area for filtration is achieved through a large flat circular membrane. With cartridge filters, the membrane is folded and pleated into a more compact design. Regardless of these differences, there are commonalities in housing designs made necessary by the requirement to avoid microbiological contamination arising from processes intended to remove or reduce microbiological contamination. All filter housings should be made from smooth "polished" materials, and where possible clamps should be used rather than screw threads where contaminants can increase in numbers. Large disc filters are hardly ever seen nowadays for production purposes. Cartridge filters predominate; the reason for this has probably more to do with marketing than with science or economics, but it is correct to say that large disc filters take longer to change, clean, and replace than cartridge filters, particularly with stacked disc combinations.

1. Disc Filters: Traditional types of large disc filter holders, if used at all for production purposes, are usually about 300 mm in diameter. The direction of fluid flow is from above the filter to below. The membrane is sandwiched between metal inlet and outlet plates equipped with the sanitary connections necessary to operate the filter. Because of the fragility of disc-type membranes, there must always be a support plate directly beneath the membrane. Support plates must be porous, often photoetched, chemically inert, and have minimal effects on flow rate. This often means an uneasy compromise. Prevention of flow restriction requires extensive void space; this acts against the plate's mechanical strength. Usually there is also a loose mesh drain plate beneath the support plate and resting on the outlet plate (Fig. 2). When serially stacked disc filters are used, each membrane requires its own support plate but there will only be one drain plate.

The whole unit is sealed by means of pressure on one or two O-rings. Where the design of the holder includes only one O-ring it is intended to serve two purposes, first to seal the inlet plate to the outlet plate and second to seal the membrane by downward compressive forces against the support and drain plates. Where the design includes two O-rings, one seals the inlet and outlet plates and the other, of a smaller diameter, sits between the membrane and the inlet plate.

Small disc filters and small single-use stacked disc filters in plastic housings are available and have the appearance of cartridge filters but consist of a series of separate membranes rather than of one continuous pleated membrane. This added complexity may make sterilization by saturated steam more difficult. Deep vacuums intended to ensure effective air removal from the filter media

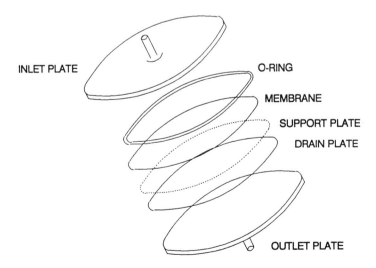

INLET PLATE   O-RING

MEMBRANE

SUPPORT PLATE

DRAIN PLATE

OUTLET PLATE

Fig. 2 Schematic representation of a disc filter.

may raise the membranes from their support screens, thus imposing an undesirable strain on the adhesion between the two. This may lead to loss of integrity. Avoidance of this risk often necessitates repeated shallow initial vacuums or long dynamic steam bleed phases prior to exposure at temperature in the autoclave.

2. Cartridge Filters: There are two major components of cartridge filters, the cartridge and the housing.

The operational part of the cartridge is the membrane, pleated to provide a significantly large surface area in a compact presentation. A cartridge filter of 5 cm diameter and 25 cm length may contain up to about 6500 cm^2 of pleated membrane surface [6]. Greater surface areas of membrane require lower applied differential pressures to achieve acceptable rates of volume flow through filters. The membrane is in most instances sandwiched between two support layers of a pleated protective nonwoven fabric (Fig. 3). This is mainly because membranes

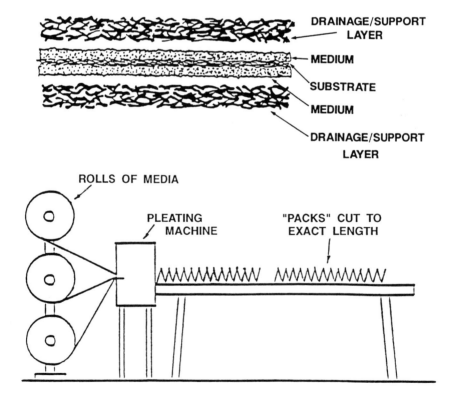

Fig. 3 Construction of pleated membranes for cartridge filters. (Courtesy of the Pall Company, Glen Cove, New York.)

are quite brittle and therefore unsuited to automated pleating. The pleated supports give a small radius of curvature to the pleated membrane rather than a sharp fold that could lead to membrane damage. The outer support layer acts also as a prefilter, protecting the membrane in another way.

The pleats are positioned between a perforated hollow tube, which comprises the inner core of the cartridge, and another perforated hollow tube (Fig. 4) or "cage," which keeps the pleats in place and forms the outer cylinder of the cartridge. The whole assembly is held together by two terminal end caps. All of the various components are bonded together in order to avoid any possibility of fluid bypassing the membrane; bonding is achieved by use of low melting point thermoplastic sealants.

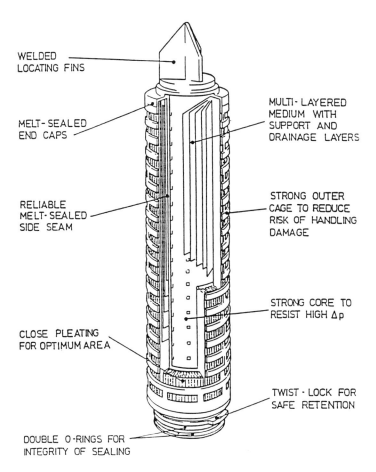

WELDED
LOCATING FINS

MELT-SEALED
END CAPS

RELIABLE
MELT-SEALED
SIDE SEAM

CLOSE PLEATING
FOR OPTIMUM AREA

DOUBLE O-RINGS FOR
INTEGRITY OF SEALING

MULTI-LAYERED
MEDIUM WITH
SUPPORT AND
DRAINAGE LAYERS

STRONG OUTER
CAGE TO REDUCE
RISK OF HANDLING
DAMAGE

STRONG CORE TO
RESIST HIGH Δp

TWIST-LOCK FOR
SAFE RETENTION

Fig. 4 Construction of a filter cartridge. (Courtesy of the Pall Company, Glen Cove, New York)

The movement of fluid across the membrane in cartridge filters is from outside to inside. When cartridges are fitted into their housings, sealing surfaces are between the end caps and adapters on the housings.

Housings may be single-cartridge housings or multi-cartridge housings. They are cylindrical, they are made of stainless steel, and all connections, etc., are designed to consider minimizing the possibility of microbiological contamination. Where the inlet and outlet ports are located at opposite ends of the housings, the term "straight-through" housing is applied; where the inlet and outlet ports are located at the same end, the term "T-type" housing is applied. The T-type housing is most suited for incorporation into rigid pipework systems.

B. Filtration of Liquids

The general case for pharmaceutical products includes sterile filtration of small-volume parenterals either in aseptic manufacture or prior to terminal sterilization, sterile filtration of ophthalmic products, and filtration of large-volume parenterals prior to terminal sterilization.

For sterile filtration of ophthalmics and small-volume parenteral products it is not unusual to find several filters mounted in series. For instance a compounded bulk product may be filtered "through the wall" from a clean area into an aseptic filling room. In these cases there are usually two filters mounted in series, one on either side of the wall. The filtrate may be fed directly to a filling machine, alternatively it may be collected in an intermediate vessel, held for a while, and then filled out. Intermediate vessels should be equipped with sterile vent filters to prevent pressure increases leading to "blow-backs."

Most large-volume parenterals are terminally sterilized, but regardless of this it is quite usual to find them being passed through a sterilizing filter prior to autoclaving. This is because of the risk of endotoxic shock from parenteral infusion of large volumes containing even only small concentrations of nonviable but still pyrogenic microbial material.

C. Filtration of Gases

Cartridge-type hydrophobic membrane filtration has largely replaced depth filtration as a means of sterilizing gases. Collection of particles from a gas stream by membrane filtration is, as with liquid filtration, a function of both sieving and other means of retention. Adsorption and electrostatic attraction are far more important to retention of particles in gas filtration than in liquid filtration. Because there are more mechanisms and interactions between pore surfaces and particles, removal of particles is more easily accomplished from gas streams than from liquids. Gases are quite satisfactorily sterilized using 0.45 µm pore size rated membranes.

Sterile filtration of gases has three main applications: first, when sterile air is required as an ingredient gas in fermentation processes; second, when gases are used for service purposes in sterile manufacture, for instance to actuate valves and to stabilize head space contents, and third, to protect the venting of sterile enclosures such as storage tanks.

Gas filters may be evaluated prior to use by the same methods used for liquid filters (see Section III below), allowing that they can be effectively dried out and sterilized without loss of the qualities being tested. Alternatively they may be evaluated by exposure to particles in a gas stream, for instance by the sodium flame test, which is also used for HEPA filters. Microbiological tests have to be considered in a somewhat different light. Leahy and Gabler [7] describe an aerosol challenge test of 10^7 *Ps. diminuta* bacteria per mL over a four-day period as an appropriate manufacturer's validation test. It would not be practical for routine use.

In-process verification of the sterility of filtered gases may be done by constantly "bleeding" off a trickle of gas through a pressure reducer on the downstream side of the sterilizing filter. The bleed may be filtered through a gelatin membrane, which should be removed daily or at other suitable intervals for incubation and examination for evidence of microbiological contamination.

III. VALIDATION AND ROUTINE CONTROL OF STERILE FILTRATION

The prime purpose of sterile filtration is to produce a sterile effluent that has not been altered as a result of the process of sterilization. Within these considerations, validation must address the performance of both the filter media and the whole filtration unit including housings, seals, connections, etc., versus its practical application. As with any other sterilization process, the continued effectiveness of sterile filtration cannot be assumed without confirmation from routine monitoring; end-product sterility testing (or testing for nonsterility) is unsuited for this purpose.

A. Validation by the Filter Manufacturer

Validation of membrane characteristics normally requires specialized techniques that lie within the expertise and experience of the membrane suppliers.

1. Extractables: Membrane filters and their housings should be chemically and biologically inert. Filter manufacturers are therefore obliged to provide evidence that minimal amounts of chemical substances are released from the materials going into their products.

Since the membrane usually presents the largest surface area of material in commercial filters, it is from membrane contamination during manufacture that most "extractables" arise. Dust particles, chemical pore formers, and solvents may be left on membranes. Wetting agents may be released from hydrophilic membranes. Indeed, Triton X-100 was at one time widely used as a wetting agent for sterilizing membranes, until it was found to be cytotoxic.

Extractables testing may be done on each individual component or material of manufacture, or on the composite assembly. The purpose of extractables testing is to determine the amount of material that can be extracted in water and in the range of solvents for which the manufacturer claims suitability. Extraction conditions should include a simulation of those processes that may affect the materials prior to use; the most obvious of these for sterilizing filters is steam sterilization. Typically, filters are autoclaved and then immersed in water or whatever solvent at 20°C and agitated for a defined period. Some extractions with volatile solvents may be done at higher temperatures and may include refluxing.

The extracts are quantified. This may be quoted directly as the weight of nonvolatile materials per filter cartridge or per unit weight or per unit of surface area, according to which is most appropriate. Alternatively, extractables may be quoted in relation to a pharmacopoeial oxidizable substances test. The primary purpose of this test is to monitor water quality, the inference being that the amount of materials extractable from the filter is no worse than the pharmacopoeial standards for water.

Biological testing may require separate extraction. All materials should meet pharmacopoeial biological safety standards. These standards for plastics require that each material be separately extracted in saline, alcohol diluted in saline, polyethylene glycol, and vegetable oil for specified conditions of time and temperature. Extracts must be tested against mice for acute systemic toxicity, against rabbits for intracutaneous reactivity, against rabbits again for pyrogens (or nowadays more likely by LAL testing for bacterial endotoxins), and against microorganisms for mutagenicity by the Ames test.

The most stringent biological test is by implantation of filter media or cartridge materials into the muscle tissue of rabbits.

None of the testing done by the manufacturers of filters can guarantee that unacceptable substances or biologically active substances are not going to be extracted into a particular pharmaceutical formulation. It is therefore incumbent upon all users of sterilizing filters to perform validation trials particular to their own applications. This usually means nonvolatile extractables and LAL testing, but it may include other methods if these do not give adequate assurance.

2. Microbial Retention: It is not common for filter users to perform microbial retention tests. In principle, microbial retention testing is quite simple; the test organism is *Pseudomonas diminuta* ATCC 19146 and the challenge is 10^7 bacteria per cm^2 of effective filtration area. The entire filtrate that has passed through the filter under test is collected on an analytical membrane; this is then incubated on an appropriate medium, and any bacteria that have passed through the test membrane are counted as colonies. The ability of the test filter to retain the challenge organism is expressed as the log reduction value (LRV) of the test filter. The LRV is defined as the $\log_{10}$ of the ratio of the number of organisms in the challenge to the number of organisms in the filtrate. Most commercial filters tested by this method yield a sterile filtrate; in these circumstances 1 is substituted in the denominator of the equation required to calculate the LRV, and the results are reported as "greater than" the LRV calculated.

Ps. diminuta is an inherently small, motile, gram-negative bacterium that was originally isolated as a contaminant of filter "sterilized" fluids. Its size, however, is not independent of nutritional and physiological factors that may be encountered in its cultivation. Smallest cell sizes occur only in the stationary phase of the organism's growth cycle. Regrettably for microbial retention testing, microbial cultures in this phase of growth also contain significant numbers of dead cells and debris. These particles that are not discernable as part of the viable microbial challenge are capable of clogging the pores of the filters under test and effectively reducing the challenge. In other phases of the growth cycle, the size of *Ps. diminuta* is larger than its quoted 0.3 μm.

Saline lactose broth is most often used for the organism's cultivation. At 30°C static incubation, *Ps. diminuta* grows as small separate single cells. In richer media, *Ps. diminuta* may grow as a pellicle; with agitation, groups of four or five cells may bind together in rosette-shaped clusters. Both of these situations are less challenging than intended.

The Health Industry Manufacturer's Association [8] has described detailed methods of performing microbial retention tests on disc- and cartridge-type sterilizing filters. In both cases it is first necessary to pass a volume of peptone water, saline, or other appropriate fluid through the filter, for two purposes: first to wet the test filter thoroughly and second to ensure that the test filter is itself sterile. The test is not considered valid unless this negative control is sterile. For disc-type filters, the challenge suspension is then passed through the membrane while maintaining a constant differential pressure of 30 psig across the membrane; for cartridge filters the standard is to maintain a flow rate of 3.86 L per min per 0.1 m^2 of effective filter area.

B. Validation and Routine Testing by the Filter User

There are certain things that must be done by filter users as part of validation before using a particular type of filter; other tests have to be done before and/or after use of each individual filter; and yet other indicators ought to be monitored throughout use of individual filters. The distinction between validation and routine monitoring is less clear for sterile filtration than for any other sterilization process.

As mentioned above, it is an obligation of the filter user to validate the sterilization processes applied to the filter. Most often sterilizing filters will be autoclaved. The effects of a particular autoclave process on the quality and quantity of extractables obtained from filters should be evaluated using the pharmaceutical fluid that is intended to be filtered. The filtrate should be demonstrated to be particle free and biologically inert; chemical extractables should not exceed the levels of contaminants allowed in the product quality specification.

The integrity of sterilizing filters is most often validated and routinely monitored by nondestructive methods. The U.S., European, and U.K. guidelines on sterile filtration refer to four methods of integrity measurement: filtration flow rate, bubble point tests, diffusion (forward flow) tests, and pressure hold tests. Each of these has its uses in determining that routinely used filters are performing to the same standards as those validated for the particular products and processes.

1. Filtration Flow Rate: In some cases the time taken to filter a specified volume of product under constant pressure may be taken as an index of filter integrity. Unduly fast filtration may be indicative of a major loss of physical integrity. Filtration flow rate is not sufficiently sensitive to detect defects in filters, which although physically quite small could contribute significantly to loss of sterility. A pinhole large enough to allow microorganisms to stream through a filter might only increase the rate of flow by as little as one mL per min; compared to, for example, an overall flow rate of 10 L per min, the effect of the pinhole on the overall time of filtration would be insignificant.

Furthermore, filtration flow rate is only useful when fluids are being filtered into intermediate vessels before filling. It is impractical where the rate of filtration is governed by the operating rate of on-line filling machines.

2. Bubble Point Test: Theoretical aspects of the bubble point test have been addressed in Section I above. The bubble point test predicts the performance of a filter by detecting the differential pressure at which a fluid is displaced by gas from the pores of a wetted filter, thus allowing capillary flow of the gas through the filter.

The classic laboratory bubble point test (Fig. 5) looks crude from a technological standpoint but is in fact very sensitive for determining the bubble point for a sample of membrane. A wetted filter element is held between support screens, and the differential pressure across the filter is gradually increased by manually adjusting a supply of compressed air. The pressure at which the first bubble appears downstream of the filter is read off from an upstream pressure gauge. Everything is dependent upon successful visual detection of the first bubble. This is not readily achievable for commercial filters because disc housings, cartridge housings, etc., prevent bubbles being seen.

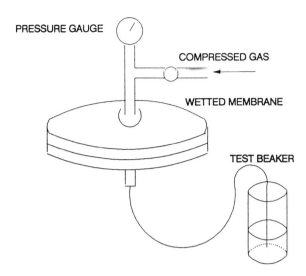

PRESSURE GAUGE

COMPRESSED GAS

WETTED MEMBRANE

TEST BEAKER

Fig. 5 Schematic representation of the bubble point test.

The bubble point test applied to commercial filters is usually an in-process test based on the flow detection. The FDA *Guideline* [1] and other regulatory statements require the test to be done before and after use. The value of doing this is to demonstrate that the filter is fit for use before filtration commences, and then to confirm that leaks or perforations or other forms of damage have not arisen during use. Automated equipment is widely used with upstream or down-stream mass or volume flow meters monitoring progress toward the bubble point. The bubble point is identified as the transition pressure at which the rate of flow of gas through the membrane abruptly changes to capillary flow. In practice this change is not as abrupt as simple theory might suggest.

Fig. 6 depicts the type of relationship that might be found between down-stream gas flow rate and upstream gas pressure in a typical in-process automated bubble point test. The transition pressure is not clearly defined. Actual bubble points (transition pressures) obtained with this type of equipment differ from theoretical bubble points calculated for the same membrane from direct mea-surement of pore size, and from laboratory-type bubble point testing.

The ideal relationship of two straight lines crossing one another can never arise because of certain unavoidable phenomena that occur during the test. First, there must always be gas flow at pressures below the bubble point; this is a result of diffusion of gas through the liquid-filled membrane (see below). Diffusional flow is proportional to the applied upstream gas pressure. The second factor is associated with the distribution of pore sizes in commercial membranes. As with

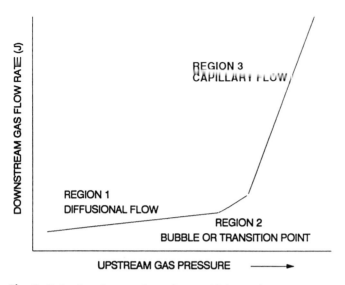

Fig. 6 Behavior of a wetted membrane with increasing gas pressure.

all manufacturing processes, perfect uniformity of pore size is not achievable in the manufacture of membrane filters. In region 2 of Fig. 6, gas is beginning to flow through the largest pores in the membrane, and flow increases as progressively smaller pores become evacuated of fluid. Automated bubble point testing equipment utilizing the principles of Fig. 6 to determine the bubble point from the transition pressure may not be effective in distinguishing membranes that have the same mean pore size but with different distributions of pore sizes (Fig. 7). Third, pores are rarely neatly cylindrical passing through the membrane by the shortest possible route. In actuality, pores follow tortuous routes through membranes and do not have uniform diameters throughout their lengths, so that pores with identical surface diameters may require quite different pressures to displace their fluid contents.

For routine control, it is unlikely that the bubble point is ever determined. It is quite usual for automated equipment to test a filter at a single pressure that is, if the validated condition is being maintained, known to be lower than the bubble point. A failure condition is flagged if the bubble point is reached at or below that set single-point pressure.

Pall and Kirnbauer [3] have identified an alternative expression of the bubble point pressure. At pressures below the bubble point, diffusional flow of gas through the membrane is proportional to the applied pressure. If the rate of gas flow per unit pressure is plotted against pressure (Fig. 8), flow will be con-

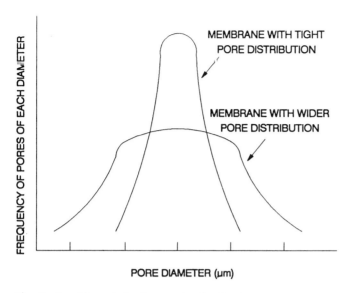

Fig. 7 Possible variation in pore size distributions.

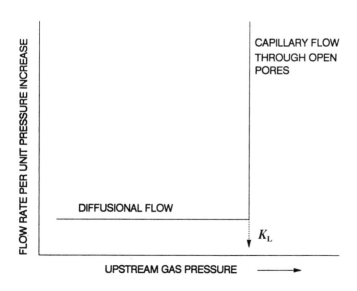

Fig. 8 Behavior of a wetted membrane with increasing gas pressure.

stant while only diffusional flow is occurring, and the transition to capillary flow will be effectively abrupt. This transition pressure is referred to as K_L.

The deficiencies and nonidealities that occur in bubble point testing should not be taken as contraindications of the usefulness of the method for in-process nondestructive filter integrity testing. It is in fact an extremely valuable in-process test. Its limitations should be understood and its value confined to comparing one filter with another of the same type.

3. *Diffusion Test*: Filter integrity may be evaluated using the fact that gas is able to flow through wetted filters by diffusion at pressures lower than the bubble point pressure. In practice, diffusion tests are automated; equipment is available to measure flow rate across filters by upstream or downstream flow meters or by upstream pressure gauges. Measurement by downstream flow meter is termed "forward flow," a term originally used by the Pall Corporation to describe their own variant of diffusion testing, now widely used to describe any type of diffusion testing regardless of location of the measuring device. Diffusion testing is done in-place, in-process, and nondestructively.

The principle of the test is that of diffusion of gases from locations where they are in high concentration (upstream of a filter) to locations where they are in low concentration (downstream of a filter). Gas will pass through a wetted membrane thus: it first dissolves in the liquid at the upstream side of the membrane, it then diffuses through the liquid phase, and it finally leaves the liquid downstream of the membrane because of the lower partial gas pressure on that side. In simple terms, we can consider membranes to be impermeable to gas, and therefore any movement of gas through a filter must be only through the liquid-filled pores. Where there is a large equivalent area of pores there will be a greater amount of diffusion than when there is only a small equivalent area of pores.

The liquid acts as a barrier to free migration of gas. The rate of diffusion of gas is brought to a steady state when the rate of diffusion of the gas into the liquid on the upstream side is just equal to the rate at which the gas is diffusing out of the membrane on the downstream side. Various steady-state conditions may exist according to pressure (the solubility of gases in liquids increases with pressure), temperature (the solubility of gases in liquids decreases with temperature but the rate of diffusion increases), and other controllable factors. The interrelationships of these factors can be predicted from Fick's laws of diffusion and the gas laws.

Fick's laws allow the rate of diffusion at steady state to be calculated from

$$J = \frac{D \cdot H \cdot P \cdot \theta}{L}$$

where J = rate of diffusional flow of the gas measured as moles of gas per unit time; D = diffusion coefficient for the gas-liquid system involved, e.g., 2×10^{-5} cm^2/s for nitrogen in water at 20°C; H = solubility coefficient for the gas-liquid system, e.g., 6.6×10^{-7} g mol/cm for nitrogen in water at 20°C; P = the upstream pressure; θ = effective area of pores (porosity or void fraction); and L = the thickness of the filter under test.

The importance of this equation is that it demonstrates that J is a linear function of the test pressure P, as long as the transition pressure between diffusive flow and capillary flow is not reached or exceeded. Other variables that must be controlled in diffusion testing include (a) the filter membrane area, because it defines the effective area of pores or void fraction; (b) the temperature, because it defines the solubility of gas in liquid; and (c) the composition of the liquid phase, because the presence of solutes affects the solubility coefficient.

As an in-process test it is usual to monitor the rate of diffusive flow at only one predetermined pressure below the bubble point. In these single-point tests, higher than normal rates of diffusional flow indicate greater than normal void fractions and probably therefore pores of greater than normal diameter (increased diffusive flow) or some perforation or damage to the filter (capillary flow). Evidence of a filter being able to hold a linear relationship between pressure and rate of diffusional flow over a range of pressures would define a more reliable measure of filter integrity but is rarely encountered in routine use. Single-point diffusion testing is recommended [8] to be done at pressures around 80% of the bubble point pressure. At pressures significantly lower than the bubble point pressure there is likely to be some difficulty in distinguishing between membranes with similar void fractions but possibly widely differing pore diameters (Fig. 9). The rate of diffusional flow from diffusion testing is best used, therefore, in conjunction with bubble point data to define validated specifications for filter integrity.

4. Pressure Hold (Pressure Decay) Test: Pressure hold tests require a wetted filter to be pressurized with gas. Further supply of gas is then shut off. The pressure decay in the filter is monitored over time and compared to predetermined standards.

The pressure hold test can be set up as a variant of the bubble point test by using a pressure slightly below the estimated bubble point. It can be set up as a variant of the diffusion test with the pressure around 80% of the bubble point pressure, or it can be set up at lower pressures around 5–10% of the bubble point pressure. The test can be done over a very short period of time or over a protracted hold time.

Pressure decay tests are mainly used as prefiltration integrity tests for cartridge filters.

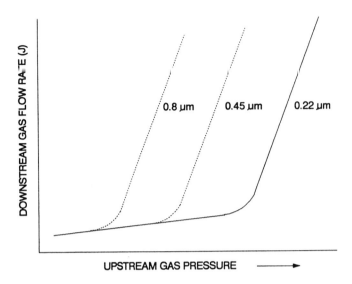

Fig. 9 Bubble points and diffusional characteristics of membranes with similar void fractions.

5. Water Penetration Test: Hydrophobic filters are in the main tested by bubble point, diffusion, or pressure decay methods based on wetting with solvents with lower surface tensions than those of the membranes. This is because the void space of the membrane will not be completely penetrated by water to allow these tests to be applicable. The main alternative solvents used in association with hydrophobic filters are aqueous solutions of isopropanol. This practice, although perfectly legitimate, introduces other problems, namely the problem of removing all of the solvent, to ensure that product coming into contact with filtered gas or air is not to be adulterated, and the problem of flammability of solvents. The water penetration (water intrusion) test is an alternative method applicable only to hydrophobic filters, which by using water rather than solvents avoids the problems described above.

The principle of the water intrusion test derives from the mercury intrusion test, which (applicable to both hydrophilic and hydrophobic membranes) is restricted to laboratory conditions. The membrane is placed in contact with the fluid (water in the case of the water penetration test, mercury in the case of the mercury intrusion test), and the pressure is increased, with the purpose of forcing the fluid into the pores. The volume of fluid forced into the pores is a measure of pore size and void space volume and thus of filter integrity.

In practice the test is done as almost a mirror image of the bubble point test. The filter housing is filled completely with water, and pressure on the upstream side is increased incrementally until water flow is seen on the downstream side (breakthrough pressure). Pore diameter is related to breakthrough pressure in the same way as it is to bubble point pressure:

$$d = -4y \cdot \frac{\cos \theta}{P}$$

This is the same equation as the bubble point equation except for the inclusion of a minus sign to compensate for the fact that the contact angle between nonwetting liquids and hydrophobic filters is greater than 90° and the cosine has therefore a negative value. In detail, d = the diameter of the pore; y = the surface tension of the liquid filling the pore; P = the breakthrough pressure; and θ = the contact angle between the liquid and the pore wall (greater than 90° for hydrophobic membranes).

In practice it is not usual to test filters to the water breakthrough pressure but, as with diffusion tests, only to some point below a breakthrough pressure derived by the filter manufacturer; breakthrough at these lower pressures may be indicative of loss of filter integrity or seal integrity failure, alternatively false failures may be caused by air pockets in the housing or residual water left in pores after steam sterilization. At pressures below breakthrough, water is forced into the pores of the filter at a rate proportional to the increase in applied pressure. If pressure is held constant below breakthrough, water penetration stabilizes to a constant rate with time, usually measured in terms of mL/10 min. This rate is typical for particular types of filter and can be used as a comparative index of filter integrity with manufacturer's values and values obtained before and after use. The rather curious denominator of 10 min is because of the really very small volumes of water that penetrate hydrophobic filters below breakthrough.

Water penetration rates are usually calculated according to the gas laws from measurement of pressure decay upstream of the filter over the whole period of testing with the gas (air) volume above the fluid held constant. They are therefore subject to temperature variations. Although the principle of the water penetration test is sound, and the avoidance of the use of potentially adulterating solvents is attractive, the low rates of water penetration calculable from only very small pressure drops within test systems have raised doubts about the robustness of the method for routine application in its contribution to the decision-making process.

6. Microbiological Monitoring: Microbiological methods of monitoring the effluent from a sterilizing filter are too insensitive to discern any but the most serious failures of the filtration system. Such failures are better detected by the nonmicrobiological in-process integrity tests described above. It is, however, normal in the application of sterile filtration to ensure that the microbiological challenge to the filter is well within the filter's sterilizing capability. Microbiological limits should be set therefore for the nonsterile challenge material; if measured numbers are high or exceed justifiable limits, prefiltration or some other means of reducing the microbial challenge should be introduced.

IV. SUMMARY OF REASONS FOR FILTRATION FAILURE

In certain circumstances sterilizing filters may allow the passage of microorganisms. It may be of value for preventing this to summarize the main reasons for the occurrence of nonsterile effluents.

(a) Incorrect assembly. Sterilizing filters must be assembled aseptically. It is difficult to legislate this except by thorough training and good supervision. The number and frequency of aseptic connections should be minimized as far as practicality dictates.

(b) Passage through defects. Filters may be flawed or defective. The defects may be within the membrane, or in the housing, or between the membrane and the housings. Routine integrity testing should be capable of revealing these types of defects through consideration of all data from bubble point, diffusion, and pressure hold tests.

(c) Passage through the membrane. The mechanism of particle retention by membrane filters is not confined to sieving. It is not therefore out of the question that there may be a coincidence of a microorganism at the bottom end of its size range and a pore at the top end of its size range. Part of the answer to this possible failure mode is for filter manufacturers to control their pore sizes within bands of only narrow variation. From the user's point of view, the challenge should be kept well within the capability of the filter.

(d) Grow-through. Microorganisms retained on a wet membrane for an extended period of time at ambient temperatures may be able to reproduce and grow through to the downstream side of the filter. This is probably more likely with air filters than with liquid filters or other gas filters. In part this is due to the time over which air filters are kept in place; in part it is due to the likelihood of moisture being carried in the airstream. It can be avoided by prefiltration and by controlling the duration of use.

REFERENCES

1. Food and Drug Administration (1987). *Guideline on Sterile Drug Products Produced by Aseptic Processing.*
2. Schroeder, H. G., and DeLuca, P. P. (1980). Theoretical aspects of sterile filtration and integrity testing. *Pharmaceutical Technology* **4**: 80–85.
3. Pall, D. B., and Kirnbauer, E. A. (1978). Bacteria removal prediction in membrane filters. In *Proceedings of 52nd Colloid and Surface Science Symposium,* University of Tennessee, Knoxville, Tennessee.

4. Leahy, T. J., and Sullivan, M. J. (1978). Validation of bacterial retention capabilities of membrane filters. *Pharmaceutical Technology* **2**: 65–75.

5. Pall, D. B., Kirnbauer, E. A., and Allen, B. T. (1980). Particulate retention by bacteria retentive membrane filters. *Colloids and Surfaces* **1**. 235–256.

6. Meltzer, T. H. (1987). *Filtration in the Pharmaceutical Industry*. New York: Marcel Dekker.

7. Leahy, T. J., and Gabler, R. (1984). Sterile filtration of gases by membrane filters. *Biotechnology and Bioengineering* **26**: 836–843.

8. Health Industry Manufacturer's Association (1982). *Microbiological Evaluation of Filters for Sterilizing Liquids*. HIMA Document No 3. Volume 4. Washington D.C.: Health Industry Manufacturer's Association.

9. Reti, A. R. (1977). An assessment of test criteria for evaluating the performance and integrity of sterilizing filters. *Bulletin of the Parenteral Drug Association* **31**: 187–199.

ANNEX 1. CALCULATING THEORETICAL PORE DIAMETERS FROM BUBBLE POINT PRESSURES

If the contact angle between liquid and membrane is zero, the pore diameter can be calculated from

$$d = \frac{4y}{P}$$

where d = pore diameter, y = surface tension of the wetting liquid, and P = bubble point pressure.

With water as the wetting liquid, the bubble point obtained with a particular membrane was 4,800 mm Hg. The surface tension of water is 72 dyn/cm. This is converted into compatible units by multiplying by a correction factor of 7.5; therefore

$$d = \frac{4 \times (72 \times 7.5)}{4,800}$$

$$d = 0.45 \ \mu m$$

With isobutanol as a wetting liquid, the bubble point obtained with another type of membrane was 4.5 psig. The surface tension of isobutanol is 1.7 dyn/cm. This is converted into compatible units by multiplying by a correction factor of 0.145; therefore

$$d = \frac{4 \times (1.7 \times 0.145)}{4.5}$$

$$d = 0.22 \ \mu m$$

8
Aseptic Manufacture

All pharmaceutical products are expected to be clean in the sense of being free from viable and nonviable particles. Aseptic manufacture is a system that has at its core a situation (aseptic filling) whereby the dosage form, product contact containers, and closures that make up the final presentation are brought together after previous stages of cleaning and sterilization. There are no cleaning or sterilization processes subsequent to aseptic filling. It is imperative therefore that the conduct of aseptic filling is such that the cleanliness and assurance of sterility of the finished product is no worse than the cleanliness and assurance of sterility of the individual components.

Current regulatory thinking (particularly with the FDA) holds that aseptic manufacture is a process of last resort. If a finished presentation is suitable for terminal sterilization, then this is the method of first choice. For instance, a heat-stable dosage form in a glass ampoule should always be considered for terminal sterilization using saturated steam. Any move toward aseptic manufacture, for example replacement of heat-stable glass ampoules by heat-sensitive plastic ampoules, should be seriously addressed and justified in the light of its benefit to the patient before any formal approach is made to a regulatory body. This is because the filling stage of aseptic manufacture is essentially a passive process of protection of the dosage form from contamination, whereas terminal sterilization is an active process of killing the contaminants within the sealed finished presentation. The degree of sterility assurance cannot be predicted for aseptic manufacture in the way that it can be predicted for terminal sterilization processes, and in truth it cannot be expected to be as good.

The major distinction between aseptic manufacture and other processes of pharmaceutical manufacture (including both nonsterile and terminally sterilized presentations) is the emphasis placed on contamination control. In general terms, the sources of potential product contamination during any form of manufacture are fivefold: (a) the environmental air; (b) the manufacturing equipment, facilities, and services; (c) the dosage form, product contact containers, and closures; (d) the personnel operating the manufacturing equipment; and (e) water and drainage.

To control these sources of contamination, the critical processes of aseptic filling are done on machines or at work stations that have been designed to protect the previously cleaned and sterilized components from contamination. These work stations or filling machines must themselves be located in contamination-protected areas. These are usually clean rooms.

The broader term "aseptic manufacture" extends beyond aseptic filling *sensu stricto* to include the systems of sterilizing the components, and the systems of providing second-level and even third-level protection to the filling stage. These controls are normally afforded by aseptic manufacture being done in rooms or suites of rooms that have been designed and constructed to facilitate thorough cleaning and to maintain cleanliness and sterility during their operation.

Aseptic manufacture is a rigorous discipline. In common with terminal sterilization processes, its success or failure cannot be evaluated from end-product testing. Facilities, equipment, and monitoring regimes are therefore critical to the success of its application.

I. APPLICATIONS OF ASEPTIC MANUFACTURE

Aseptic manufacture has diverse applications. It is in use with liquid and solid sterile parenteral and ophthalmic dosage forms in simple and complex presentations including glass ampoules, rubber-sealed glass vials, plastic ampoules, prefilled glass syringes, etc. The form of presentation may be single-dose or it may be multi-dose. There are many heat-stable dosage forms in heat-stable presentations that are aseptically filled rather than being terminally sterilized. Past regulatory thinking has permitted this practice, although it is now severely frowned upon.

In some circumstances the decision to fill aseptically or to sterilize terminally must address more complex sterility-related issues than product stability. Consider, for example, the transfer and admixture of a small-volume pharmaceutically active dosage form from a glass vial into a large-volume bagged infusion fluid. The most widely used approach is to use a sterile syringe to withdraw the dosage form from the vial and inject it into the infusion fluid via a septum. Some presentations are now available whereby the contents of a vial may be directly injected into an infusion fluid bag without the need for the two syringe-mediated aseptic transfers. These involve specifically adapted infusion fluid bags and plastic-modified vials. The modified vials cannot be terminally sterilized. The question to be addressed is which is of greater risk or benefit to the patient, a terminally sterilized product that must be aseptically transferred twice at point of use or an aseptically manufactured product that need only be transferred once?

Ophthalmic products, eyedrops in single-dose and multi-dose presentations, and eye ointments in multi-dose presentations are aseptically manufactured. So also are some other topical products. Glass eyedrop bottles are now less common than plastic ones; aluminum ointment tubes are still more commonly used for sterile products than plastic tubes. Plastic caps are almost universally used.

Many aseptically manufactured presentations are formulated to include preservatives. These may serve one or both of two purposes. First, they contribute an active antimicrobial process following on from aseptic filling. This can be important to affording maximum patient protection. For a product to be potentially infective, microorganisms must not only contaminate it, they must also be able to survive in it. Aseptic manufacture can never provide a 100% guarantee against contamination, but preservatives may prevent the imperfections of aseptic manufacture having serious consequences. The second purpose for including preservatives is particular to multi-dose presentations where their purpose is to prevent proliferation of any microorganisms that might contaminate the product over repeated intrusions in use. It must be emphasized that preservatives are not included as an alternative to product protection during manufacture. The standards of protection and control during aseptic manufacture of preserved and nonpreserved formulations must be the same.

II. SYSTEMS OF ASEPTIC MANUFACTURE

An integrated system of controls and protective measures is essential to the success of aseptic manufacture.

It is generally agreed that the most critical operation within aseptic manufacture is the aseptic filling stage. At the point of fill, the dosage form is at most risk of contamination from environmental air-borne microorganisms while it is being transferred from one form of closed containment to another. This stage of aseptic manufacture must be located in a clean room and should have some further form of localized protection from air-borne contamination.

The product may also become contaminated by surface-to-surface transfer of microorganisms from personnel and the manufacturing equipment itself. Cleanliness of manufacturing equipment is therefore imperative. Effective cleaning and decontamination procedures are therefore a necessary part of integrated aseptic manufacture.

It is also essential for equipment to be maintained in a state of cleanliness and sterility between clean-downs. In unprotected environments, contamination by air-borne microorganisms is inevitable. It is normal therefore to house aseptic filling equipment in areas that are protected from the general contaminated natural environment (clean rooms).

Movement of personnel, components, equipment, and services in and out of protected areas needs also to be controlled if the protective barriers are to be effective in preventing contamination. Many of these necessary intrusions can be brought into the protected area via some form of decontamination or sterilization process, for instance via a double-ended autoclave. Personnel cannot be effectively decontaminated in these ways but must be dressed in sterilized garments that prevent skin-borne and hair-borne microorganisms and respiratory and digestive activities from contaminating the protected area, the manufacturing equipment, or any component of the finished presentation. Personnel must be educated and disciplined in the specific techniques of working in aseptic areas, and specific localized protection should be given to manual operations to reduce the dependency on knowledge, experience, and skills.

The separate and independent components of an effective system of aseptic manufacture overlap rather than abut against one another. Momentary failure of any one system does not necessarily compromise product sterility. Nonetheless, good assurance of avoidance of contamination can only be obtained from knowledge that each system is capable of performing as it ought to perform (validation) and that it continues to operate effectively in routine use (routine monitoring).

A. Contamination—Prevention and Control

1. Environmental Air: Microorganisms are ubiquitous in unprotected environments. Air is not a milieu that supports the growth of microorganisms, but it always carries a contaminant microflora of mainly desiccation-resistant microorganisms borne on dust, skin-flakes, and other forms of particulate matter. The only practical method of decontaminating air is by filtration.

The type of filter used for decontaminating air supplies to aseptic manufacturing is the high efficiency particle air (HEPA) filter. HEPA filters are made from glass fiber paper corrugated into pleats over aluminum separator sheets (Fig. 1). The glass fiber matrix captures particles of submicron dimensions by impaction, interception, and electrostatic forces. It is little affected by humidity and has minimal resistance to airflow. The filter element is mounted in a wood, steel, or laminate frame by means of an adhesive bonding agent that gives a rigid structure when set hard. The downstream sides of HEPA filters are fitted with rubber gaskets.

HEPA filters are classified according to their efficiency with respect to preventing penetration of submicron particles. They range from 95% efficiency to 99.999%. Filter suppliers usually quote efficiencies in relation to one or both of two test methods:

(a) The sodium flame test. This test is based on a challenge of sodium chloride particles (size range, 0.02 to 2 μm with a median diameter of 0.6 μm). Any particles passing through a filter are detected by flame photometry.

(b) The oil aerosol test. This test is commonly called the DOP test after dioctyl phthallate, which was the originally used principal oil source.

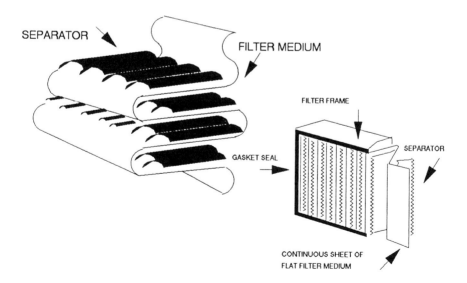

Fig. 1 Construction of a HEPA filter.

Dioctyl phthallate is not now used for this purpose because of a risk to operator health. An aerosol of mineral oil is now used. It is provided from generators that heat the oil and then vaporize it by entrainment in an inert gas stream. The particle size range is from 0.1 to 1.25 μm with a median diameter of 0.3 μm. Aerosol particles passing through a filter are detected with an aerosol photometer.

Installation of HEPA filters into their housings in an air-handling system depends very much on the design of the housing. Some filters are simply sealed against a flat steel housing fitted with ledges to support the filter. Compression of the gasket is by a clamping mechanism at the back of the filter. Other filter housings may have a "knife edge" to seal against the gasket the better to prevent channelling of unfiltered air between the filter and the housing.

HEPA filters are expensive and delicate. Three stages of filtration are usually used in connection with aseptic manufacture. These are prefilters, primary HEPA filters, and terminal HEPA filters. Of these it is only terminal HEPA filters that are mandatory, but in practice the extra filters significantly extend the operational life of the terminal filters, make maintenance of the terminal filters considerably easier, and reduce the risk of contamination arising from pinhole or other minor filter damage. Use of primary HEPA filters also simplifies the decision-making process in the event of damage to terminal filters being discovered only after the protected area has been used for product manufacture.

Rooms provided with HEPA-filtered air are termed clean rooms.

The layout of a typical air handling system serving an aseptic filling room or clean room is depicted in Fig. 2. A primary bank of HEPA filters is usually situated in a plant room physically separated but not remote from the aseptic manufacturing facility.

Prefilters to protect the primary HEPAs are attached to the air-inlet face and should meet a specification of not less than 80% efficiency. Prefilters should also be fitted on the outlet side of the air handling unit downstream of the chamber in which recirculating and fresh air "makeup" are mixed (Fig. 2). Primary HEPAs should be specified at 99.97% or 99.99% efficiency.

Terminal HEPAs should be located in the air supply ducts as close as possible to their point-of-use exit grilles. For aseptic filling rooms they should be specified at 99.997% efficiency. They may be set in one of two types of housing, front-withdrawal or back-withdrawal, depending on the mechanism for removal and replacement. Back-withdrawal HEPAs can be removed from outside the protected environment; front-withdrawal types have to be removed via the protected environment itself. Neither type is suited to removal and replacement with the area remaining sufficiently protected for operation, but front-withdrawal is preferable because it leaves the duct work intact and not subject to contamination from unprotected service voids during removal.

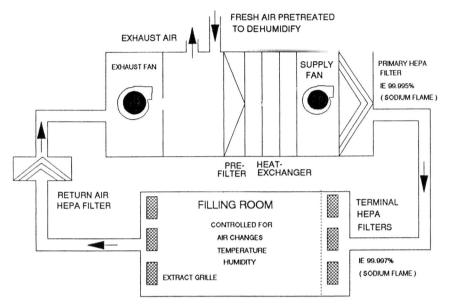

Fig. 2 Layout of a typical air handling system.

Housings for terminal HEPAs should have airtight seals to the ceiling behind the grilles or diffusers. The sealing of the HEPA filter should be on the air-inlet side of front-withdrawal HEPAs and on the air-outlet side of back-withdrawal HEPAs. Filter housings should be equipped with an access port behind the filter to allow access of smoke for validation purposes (see below).

Although environmental air is itself a source of potential contamination, it can also, once filtered, be used to prevent contamination. Microorganisms are not equipped with any means of moving in an airstream; significantly, they cannot "swim upstream" against a positive air pressure.

Pressure differentials have widespread use in aseptic manufacture to protect critical operations and critical areas from adjacent areas of lower criticality. The second protective effect that can be exerted by air is a "sweeping" one. High-velocity filtered air (greater than 90 ft/min), termed laminar flow, has the capability of protecting critical operations by sweeping particles and microorganisms away from the sensitive area. Vertical and horizontal laminar flow units are available, classified according to the direction of airflow. Laminar flow is widely used for localized protection in aseptic manufacture, for instance at point of fill in aseptic filling, over aseptic manipulations involving personnel and numerous other situations.

2. Manufacturing Equipment, Facilities and Services: Microorganisms can survive, and indeed proliferate, on the surfaces of seemingly inert objects like walls, floors, and machine parts. The presence of even small amounts of organic materials, oils, or greases may increase their resistance to naturally inimical forces present in the environment. Unprotected manufacturing facilities and equipment inevitably become contaminated by deposition of microorganisms from the environmental air, and by surface to surface transfer from personnel. In facilities protected from the general environment by the provision of filtered air, pressure differentials, and perhaps laminar flow, surfaces that are decontaminated ought not to become recontaminated. Cleaning and decontamination of equipment is a primary and major system of contamination control.

Demountable product contact machine parts for aseptic filling are best cleaned outside the filling room. It is not a good idea to situate wash-bays in critical areas. Water is always a potentially major source of microbiological contamination, and water-borne microorganisms, particularly *Pseudomonas* spp, are notable for their ability to increase in numbers in circumstances where nutrients are in very low concentration, and to be able to use the most unlikely compounds to support growth. Returning these parts to the filling room should preferably be via a terminal sterilization process, or after decontamination with an appropriate disinfectant via an interlock, air lock, or hatch designed to prevent loss of air pressure in the protected area and to facilitate disinfection.

Fixed equipment, walls, floors, and ceilings can only periodically be thoroughly cleaned down and decontaminated. There are only two approaches to cleaning acceptable for aseptic manufacturing areas, wet wiping or a vacuum cleaner equipped with a HEPA filtered exhaust.

Vacuum cleaners, however, are only suited to areas outside aseptic filling rooms because of their relative inefficiency of collection of smaller particles [1], leaving wet wiping with disinfectants as the "standard" method used for cleaning filling rooms.

The choice of disinfectants is never easy. Cross-contamination of the product with disinfectant traces is to be avoided at all costs. All disinfectants brought into aseptic filling rooms either for major clean downs or for routine use should be filtered into sterilized containers via 0.22 μm pore size sterilizing filters. It is also important for disinfectants to be rotated to prevent selection of resistant populations of contaminants. Alcohols (ethanol or isopropanol) are well suited to aseptic filling room use, as also are some proprietary disinfectants such as chlorhexidine that are specifically manufactured for such purposes. Periodically the whole aseptic manufacturing area may be fumigated; formaldehyde has been in common use but is declining due to its potential risk to the health of personnel who must work in fumigated areas.

Services should be provided from outside aseptic filling rooms, either by routing within the fabric of the surrounding walls, floors, or ceilings, or from adjoining less critical areas of the aseptic manufacturing facility. Light fittings should be fitted flush to walls or ceilings to prevent unnecessary uncleanable surfaces. Water should be avoided. Compressed air should be filtered through 0.22 μm pore size hydrophobic sterilizing filters.

3. Dosage Forms and Product-Contact Components: The object of aseptic manufacture is to bring a sterile dosage form and the finished presentation's presterilized product contact components together without contaminating them. Confidence of their sterility is of major importance. This means validated sterilization processes and low levels of microbiological contamination prior to their sterilization.

Parenteral solid dosage forms, e.g., antibiotics, are most usually delivered as the sterile drug substance from primary fermentation and conversion operations to secondary aseptic manufacturing facilities. They may or may not be blended aseptically with other sterile excipients before aseptic filling. Blending should be considered as an aseptic process and be subject to all of the normal constraints. Entry into the aseptic filling room should be via an interlock, air lock, or hatch designed to prevent pressure loss in the protected area. Interlocks may incorporate some form of decontamination of the sealed container in which the dosage form is delivered, for instance ultra-violet irradiation, disinfectant bathing, or peracetic acid decontamination.

Liquid formulations should be prepared in an area that is as clean as possible. Water for parenteral products should be of pharmacopoeial *Water for Injection* quality. Mixing vessels and other equipment should be cleaned and disinfected. It is normal for these areas to be provided with filtered air from HEPA filters of somewhat lower efficiencies than those providing protection to aseptic filling rooms. Sterilization of liquid products should be by filtration through 0.22 μm sterilizing filters directly into the aseptic filling room. Two filters in series are often used; the first of these is nominally to protect the integrity of the aseptic filling room, and the second to sterilize. In practice one filter is sufficient for sterilization; two mounted in series simplifies the decision-making process in the event of one but not both filters failing post-use integrity testing.

Filtered sterile dosage forms may be collected in sealed vessels in the aseptic filling room for subsequent connection to the filling machine, or the filter outlet may be connected directly to the filling machine.

Product contact components should be washed and sterilized into aseptic filling rooms. Glass vials are commonly passed through a combined washer/dry heat tunnel connecting unprotected receiving areas to the aseptic filling room. In older or low-volume operations, glass components may be dry heat sterilized in ovens. Rubber stoppers and aluminum ointment tubes are preferably sterilized into aseptic filling areas via double-ended washer/autoclaves. Radiation or ethylene oxide sterilized product contact components like ointment tube caps and eyedrop caps should be introduced via an interlock as described for solid dosage forms. Product contact gases for sparging or over-pressurizing should be sterilized by passage through 0.22 μm pore size hydrophobic sterilizing filters.

Any storage of sterile dosage forms or sterilized components in aseptic filling rooms should be in sealed containers, and these should be afforded additional localized filtered air or laminar flow protection to prevent their contents becoming contaminated when they are opened.

4. *Personnel*: A normal healthy individual sheds about ten million or 6^{-14} g of skin scales daily. About 10% of these carry microorganisms such as *Staphylococcus* and *Propionibacterium*. Some of these may be pathogenic. In a normal population, 5 to 30% of individuals may carry *Staphylococcus aureus* in their noses and 2 to 5% may carry *Streptococcus pyogenes* in their throats. Microorganisms may also contaminate wounds and skin infections. Poor personal hygiene may permit transfer of faecal organisms on the hands.

There are five considerations given to prevention and control of contamination from personnel sources: (a) training (knowledge and practice), (b) medical screening, (c) control of access, (d) containment of the individual, and (e) protection of critical operations.

Untrained individuals should not be allowed to enter aseptic filling rooms nor attempt aseptic manipulations associated with product manufacture. Training should address an understanding of the sources, routes, and control systems relating to microbiological contamination and should concentrate on developing dexterity with respect to the specific techniques of aseptic operations. Personnel can disseminate microbial aerosols even when standing or sitting still, but the rate of dissemination increases dramatically with movement. More people in an area means more dissemination.

Individuals with medical conditions that may lead to abnormally high shedding or dissemination of microorganisms should not be chosen to work in aseptic filling rooms. Conditions include excema, psoriasis, styes and boils, coughs, colds, and hay fever.

It is personnel with symptomatic conditions who must be screened out of aseptic work; the large proportion of the population who are nonsymptomatic nondisseminating carriers of pathogenic microorganisms are no more a risk than other healthy individuals. Some aseptic manufacturing operations bar nonsymptomatic carriers of *Staphylococcus* and *Streptococcus* from critical operations. This is strangely illogical, since nonsterility is a condition that can result from contamination by any microorganism, and pathogens are no more significant than nonpathogens.

Access of personnel to aseptic filling rooms should be via a defined route, through a series of at least two changing rooms progressively meeting higher standards of cleanliness, and against a pressure differential.

The principal method of protecting aseptic filling rooms from contamination by personnel is through the provision of effective containment of their microflora within protective clothing. Personnel should never be allowed to change directly from street clothes (particularly outdoor footwear) into aseptic filling room garments. Personal clothing is usually a greater source of microbiological contamination, and therefore a greater microbiological challenge to aseptic area protective clothing, than clean skin. Protective clothing to be worn in aseptic filling rooms should cover as much of the operator's body as possible. This means head-to-toe overall garments fitting snugly at the neck, wrists and ankles, dedicated footwear, gloves, face masks, and glasses. All protective clothing should itself be supplied sterile, sterilized or effectively decontaminated before use in aseptic filling rooms.

Protective garments should not shed particles; this requirement excludes natural fibers. A variety of woven and unwoven, calendered and uncalendered polyesters and nylons are available.

One significant decision in the choice of protective garments is between so-called breathable and nonbreathable fabrics. The breathable fabrics are permeable to air (and by that fact also to some extent permeable to microrganisms) and more comfortable to wear than nonbreathable fabrics. Nonbreathable garments are less comfortable to wear (body moisture is retained within the garments), and gases may accumulate within the garments, causing first a ballooning effect that may impede manual dexterity and second a pumping out of air and microorganisms when sufficient pressure has built up. If nonbreathable garments are chosen, it is recommended that the ankles be left loose to allow this discharge to take place in the least hazardous area of the filling room.

The fourth means of avoiding contamination from personnel sources is by localized protection of critical operations that necessitate manual intervention. This includes point of fill and other operations like connecting and disconnecting feed lines, loading rubber plugs into hoppers, taking samples for quality control checks, etc. The issue to address in connection with localized protection is the extent to which it should be applied. There are two methods: (a) total containment in an isolator or glove-box, and (b) protection by means of laminar flow filtered air.

Total containment of critical operations in isolators or glove boxes is localized protection at its most severe. These systems totally separate the operator from the process. They are quite commonly used in the nuclear industry and for handling highly toxic substances, carcinogens, and pathogens.

But for these purposes the onus is on protection of the operator from the product and therefore they work at a negative pressure relative to the general environment.

Isolators for aseptic operations work at positive pressures relative to the general environment. Up-to-date isolator technologies are most often based on containment within flexible transparent PVC "tents." Sterilization of internal surfaces is by peracetic acid or hydrogen peroxide fumigation. Positive pressures are obtained by externally mounted pumps delivering and exhausting air through HEPA filters. Access for manipulations may be through glove ports or through "half-suits." The difficulty with isolators is how to get the product and components intended for aseptic filling in and out of the isolator. With flexible film manual work stations this can be resolved by bringing materials to the isolator in special containers that can be aseptically connected to entry ports. The situation is rather more difficult with high-speed industrial filling lines; some compromise of integrity of the isolator is unavoidable.

By and large the method of choice for localized protection during aseptic manufacture is by laminar flow filtered air. The principal of laminar flow is to maintain the sterility of a work area by continuously purging it with unidirectional filtered air moving along parallel flow lines. Laminar flow technology and aseptic manufacture have become so closely identified that the two terms have almost become synonymous. Since its introduction in 1961, laminar flow technology has led to a progressive expansion of high-speed aseptic manufacture and of the available range of aseptically filled pharmaceutical products.

Very small particles such as those that carry microbiological contamination (usually in the range of 8 to 14 μm in diameter) are not heavy enough to fall to ground level under gravitational forces alone. Instead they remain in air currents and move around as the air eddies.

Particles generated upstream of exposed products in aseptic filling rooms, or particles caught in regions of turbulent air, may be swept onto and into the product. The action of laminar flow (usually understood to mean an air velocity of around 90 ft/min) is to sweep across an area without creating turbulence or regions of dead air. In the event of a microbial or particulate contaminant being introduced into the laminar flow protected area, whether by having been carried in or having been generated there, the high-velocity unidirectional airflow carries it quickly away.

The big advantage of laminar flow over containment is access. Personnel can easily gain access to the area in which their intervention is necessary. Product and components can be conveyed into laminar flow protected areas without having to pass through complex barriers. Nonetheless these advantages can only be achieved through very careful application. Figure 3 illustrates a horizontal laminar flow work station. This type of application may be used for localized protection of manual operations like making and breaking aseptic connections or storage of machine parts or vial stoppers after sterilization but before loading into the filling machine hopper. This type of work station is also commonly seen in laboratory applications. Quite simply, the work station draws air from the general environment and forces it through a HEPA filter and out over the work area via a diffuser. The diffuser serves two purposes, first to protect the HEPA filter face from physical or chemical (spraying with a disinfectant, for instance)

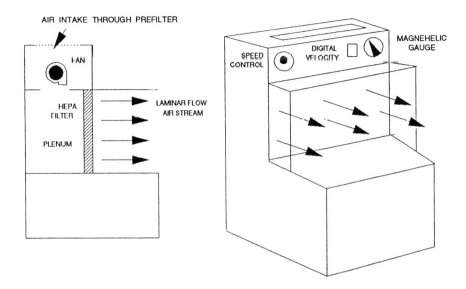

Fig. 3 Horizontal laminar flow work station.

damage by the operator, and second to ensure laminarity of air movement (Fig. 4).

Figure 5 illustrates a vertical laminar flow canopy such as might be used for localized protection of a filling machine or the off-loading station from a sterilizer. Fixed or portable versions of this type of unit are available and have a wide application in aseptic manufacture.

The precise location of portable units must be defined. Laminar flow units, although creating a protected environment within their confines, may themselves create turbulence and dead air in the room in which they are situated and into which they exhaust. This may create a secondary source of contamination. The airflow patterns around laminar flow units relative to fixed air exit registers, screening, and other equipment in a room cannot be predicted. Empirical evidence from smoke pattern studies is necessary to be confident of their effectiveness.

In the early days of laminar flow, the idea of entire rooms being protected by laminar flow was greeted with enthusiasm. They are now rarely found in connection with aseptic filling. They are far more expensive to construct than conventional turbulent flow clean rooms, because of the need for more filters and greater engineering capabilities to move a lot of air at high velocity. Moreover, a horizontal laminar flow wall provides unidirectional air flow only as far as the first work station. Thereafter it is no different from a conventional clean

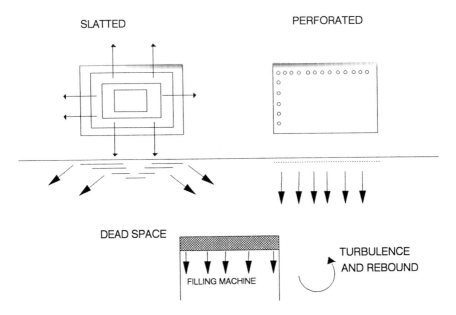

Fig. 4   Effects of different types of diffusor.

room.   Vertical laminar flow rooms do not share this problem, but inevitably they protect a greater area than is necessary.   The same effect can be created at less cost by localized vertical laminar flow canopies situated only over the critical operations.

5. Water and Drainage: Water is a potential source of microbiological contamination that cannot be excluded from aseptic manufacture.   Its control becomes complicated by the variety of purposes for which it may be used and the various types of distribution system that may be encountered.   Identifiable potential sources of contamination from water in aseptic manufacturing facilities include: (a) "ingredient" water for sterile products, (b) water supplies for equipment and component cleaning, (c) water supplies to laundries, (d) water supplies for hand washing, and (e) steam supplies to autoclaves.

The pharmacopoeias deal with ingredient water of two types, *Purified Water* and *Water for Injection*.   The principal difference in biological quality between the two types of water is that *Water for Injection* is specified to be pyrogen-free (less than 0.25 Eu of bacterial endotoxin per mL).   Only water of *Water for Injection* quality may be used to dissolve, dilute, or compound parenteral products, because endotoxins may pass through 0.22 μm sterilizing filters.   Control of bacterial endotoxins is achieved in the first instance through control of microbiological contamination.

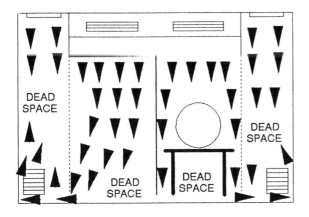

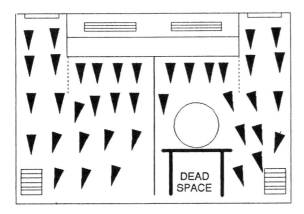

Fig. 5 Vertical laminar flow canopy (showing smoke patterns for full- and half-length curtains).

The pharmacopoeias restrict the methods by which *Water for Injection* may be prepared to distillation and to reverse osmosis. The nature of the distillation process dictates that freshly distilled water must be sterile and (except in the case of some systems failures) pyrogen free.

The molecular dimensions of bacterial endotoxins are too large to pass through reverse osmosis membranes, and therefore the process is permitted by the pharmacopoeias for production of *Water for Injection*. However, the outlet water from reverse osmosis units can easily become microbiologically contaminated by formations of films or slimes downstream of the membranes. At least two microbiological problems may be encountered with reverse osmosis. First, microbiological films may slough off into the water at unpredictable intervals or as a result of disinfection; second, these films are peculiarly resistant to disinfection and once formed may be very difficult to eradicate.

Ingredient water should be used immediately or stored under controlled conditions. Large sterile production facilities use stainless steel storage and distribution loops that keep water in continuous turbulent motion at temperatures above 80°C. All water contact surfaces should be smooth and continuous to prevent accumulation of nutrients, and the system should be designed to allow frequent draining, flushing, and sanitizing (preferably by steam at 120°C). Mains should be sloped to allow complete drainage, and "deadlegs" should be avoided; where this is impossible they should be kept as short as possible (as a rule of thumb, less than six times the diameter of the piping). Stored water should be kept under a blanket of inert gas such as nitrogen, and tanks should be provided with air filters to allow venting as water is drawn off.

Water of *Water for Injection* and *Purified Water* qualities has other applications in addition to its use as ingredient water. For instance, the final rinse water for washed product contact components and machine parts should be of no lesser quality than ingredient water. Purified water from 80°C loops is best used for machine washing, but 80°C is an unacceptably high temperature for human contact in manual operations. For these purposes water may be drawn from the high-temperature circulatory loop via local heat exchangers. However, these are prone to microbiological contamination; an alternative approach is to run a lower temperature loop (e.g., at 40°C) for these purposes. It is advisable to raise the temperature of 40°C ring mains to 80°C overnight each night to avoid buildup of microbiological contaminants.

At any moment all of the water in an aseptic manufacturing facility must be in the product, in the distribution system, or passing through the drains. Serious measures must be taken to ensure that drainage systems do not become sources of microbiological contamination and proliferation.

All equipment drains should have air breaks of a few inches separating them from floor drains. Larger air breaks do not necessarily give more assurance against drains causing contamination. Splashing from water falling greater distances may lead to the formation of microbial aerosols, which may then contaminate exposed product or manufacturing equipment. Further avoidance of splashing may be facilitated by use of conical tun dishes to channel falling water into floor drains.

Floors of preparation areas where water spillage is inevitable should be constructed "true" to avoid puddles and should have a slope of about 1:50 to a flush fitting floor drain. Floor drains are best kept as dry as possible to avoid microbial proliferation. The most effective method of sanitizing drains is by heated traps. These are heating elements capable of boiling water located in the U-bend beneath floor or sink drains. They are normally operated by timing devices to work only when there is water in the drain.

B. Typical Facility Design

At first glance it might seem that the term aseptic manufacturing facility is synonymous with the term clean room. It is not. Although aseptic filling is always
done in a clean room, the clean room is only one component of a complex of barrier systems that make up an aseptic manufacturing facility.

At the heart of aseptic manufacture is the filling machine or filling station
itself; the point of fill is thought to be the most critical location to exercise contamination control. The USP recommends a double barrier concept of contamination control, with the primary barrier toward prevention of microbiological
contamination being some sort of localized protection around this region. The
clean room (aseptic filling room) in which the filling machine is located should
constitute the secondary barrier. In practice there are usually far more layers of
protection offered to the point of fill.

Figure 6 diagrammatically represents the successive series of barriers to
contamination that exist in typical aseptic manufacturing facilities.

(a) The first layer of protection is outside the plant itself. The condition of
this area may contribute to contamination control. It is usually not thought
desirable for earth banks to abut directly against the external walls of the
facility nor for pools of stagnant water to lie in the close periphery. Many
aseptic manufacturing facilities prohibit broken soil created by building
activities to be left uncovered close to the external walls.

(b) The incoming warehouse is the first layer offering protection by a
physical barrier, the facility walls. Apart from the facts that warehouses

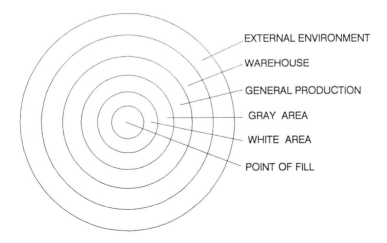

EXTERNAL ENVIRONMENT

WAREHOUSE

GENERAL PRODUCTION

GRAY AREA

WHITE AREA

POINT OF FILL

Fig. 6 Layers of protection to aseptic filling.

can be kept reasonably clean, and that pest control systems can be exercised in warehouses, the protection against contamination afforded by this layer is minimal.

(c) Even in facilities dedicated wholly to aseptic products there will be some form of general production, for instance packing sterile sealed containers for shipping. The third layer of protection is this general production area. Pest control systems must be more effective than in open-bayed warehouses. All staff can be routed through the general production area via first level changing procedures that require external street clothing to be replaced by simple factory overalls, which may range from a simple smock over street clothes to a complete change into company uniform and shoes. This is the last region within the facility that should be considered as a public area. Further progress toward the aseptic filling room should only be allowed to trained personnel.

(d) The first layer offering significant protection to aseptic manufacturing should only be enterable via a changing area requiring personnel to put on shoe covers, head covers and dedicated overalls. This part of an aseptic manufacturing facility is often, but not universally, referred to as a "gray" area. Typically it is the part of the facility where actives and excipients are dispensed and mixed, and where machine parts and components are cleaned and prepared for entry into the aseptic filling room or "white" area. Importantly, the gray areas must be maintained at a higher air pressure than the surrounding parts of the facility. Air pressure must be carefully balanced in aseptic manufacturing suites to ensure that there is a cascade of pressure differentials from the most to the least critical operations (Fig. 7). Best practice is for all personal clothing or general factory uniform clothing to be removed on entering the gray areas. Aseptic underwear may be provided to wear beneath gray area nonsterile overalls.

(e) The white area, clean room, or aseptic filling room should be sealed off from other areas, for access of product, components and personnel. Direct access that is not via some form of interlock is not permitted. Personel access to the white area may or may not be via a gray area. If it is not via a gray area, personnel should not be permitted to change directly from general factory attire into aseptic area clothing.

(f) The final zone of protection is the localized protection given to point-of-fill and to manual processes conducted within the filling room.

The interrelationships between standards of cleanliness and activities needed for gray areas and those of white areas are critical to the successful operation of aseptic manufacturing facilities.

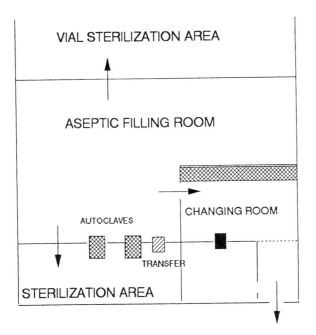

Fig. 7 Cascade of differential pressures in aseptic manufacture.

1. Gray Areas: White areas are not islands. Materials are moved in and out of white areas, and personnel enter and leave white areas. All such movements risk compromising the aseptic status of the white area. In practice these risks are minimized by the gray areas, which bridge the distance between nonsterile and aseptic conditions. Gray areas are usually classified to Clean Room Standards (see below), most often within Class 10,000 in the nonoperational condition, which means in brief less than 10,000 particles of 0.5μm diameter or greater per ft^3. This places clear engineering demands with respect to the use of HEPA filters, the number of air changes per hour, and the maintenance of positive pressure differentials.

Sundry services must be provided to the white areas via the gray areas. The most obvious of these are product dispensing and compounding. Liquid sterile products are passed into the aseptic filling room via sterilizing filters. The microbiological challenge to these filters is effectively minimized by these activities taking place under controlled conditions. This area within the gray zone may be physically separated or otherwise from equipment and component preparation areas. The risk of having these two sets of gray area operations situated too close to one another is that of contamination from water sources of differing qualities. Up-to-date facilities may use equipment that combines component washing and sterilization into one process. Irrespective of this, the loading ends of autoclaves, ovens, and tunnels leading into the aseptic filling room are located in gray areas. Access to sterilizers for maintenance and repair is not allowed from inside the white areas.

Personnel wishing to gain access to the white area must pass through a dedicated changing room. These should be supplied with air of the same quality as white areas, but they are strictly speaking gray areas. It is preferable for the white changing rooms to vent air to gray corridors or some other gray area physically separated from the gray areas in which product and components are exposed. The white changing room should not be accessible directly from the general factory environment.

These changing areas are the most likely route of entry for microbiological contamination into aseptic filling rooms. The doors leading into changing rooms and those from the changing rooms to the aseptic filling room should be interlocked in such a manner that only one set of doors can be opened at one time. In some societies safety considerations preclude this type of interlock and warning lights or alarms may be used to supplement personnel disciplines. Other features of white changing areas are step-over benches (boot barriers), hand-wash stations, and hot-air hand driers. The purpose of the step-over bench is to segregate the areas in which only designated sterilized (or sanitized) footwear may be worn from the rest of the aseptic manufacturing facility, which has less stringent footwear requirements. The hand-wash station should be provided with elbow- or foot-operated taps. Water should be provided in the temperature range of 45 to 55°C, and potential contamination from water drainage should be given special consideration. In some aseptic manufacturing facilities the risk of contamination from this source has led to a total ban on water from aseptic filling room changing areas. This is probably best practice but places high demands on discipline with regard to hand washing at earlier stages in the progression of personnel from the general factory through gray changing areas.

Last but not least, best practice is for aseptic changing rooms to be equipped with horizontal laminar flow protection, providing a gradient of air cleanliness from the filter bank situated at the cleanest end (access to the aseptic filling room) of the room to exit registers at the entrance.

Provision of aseptic area garments to changing rooms must be given serious consideration. Unless presterilized garments are being provided through transfer hatches, laundries should be situated in the gray areas adjacent. Washing machines should be of double-ended barrier types and should incorporate facilities for integral disinfectant rinsing and drying.

2. White Areas: The pressure differential between the white area and adjacent areas should be no less than 1.5 mm (0.05 in) water gauge. There must be no less than 20 air changes per hour, and the balance between recycled and fresh air makeup should be around 9:1.

Aseptic filling rooms are invariably required to be Class 100 clean rooms. Most often they are turbulent flow (conventional) clean rooms, but some facilities may operate laminar flow clean rooms. With conventional clean rooms HEPA filtered air is introduced into the room through registers situated in the ceilings or at high levels on the walls and leaves the room through low level exit registers (Fig. 8). The effects of conventional clean rooms are dilution and filtration. The air becomes thoroughly mixed within the room, and particular attention must be paid to avoid areas of dead air. Laminar flow clean rooms (described above) are more costly and are not frequently seen in connection with aseptic manufacture.

Within the filling room, all aseptic manipulations and process stages requiring exposure of the dosage form or product contact components should be protected by localized laminar flow drawing air from the Class 100 environment. The importance of this protection is not in the sterility of the air but in the sweeping effect of the air.

3. Layout: The design of aseptic manufacturing facilities and the layout of the various functional operations relative to the need for proximity and the need to maintain asepsis is highly complex and product specific. The simplest case is one of a single aseptic filling room with wholly dedicated gray areas and other services; more often several filling operations may be clustered together in one filling room, or several filling rooms may be serviced through one combined gray area.

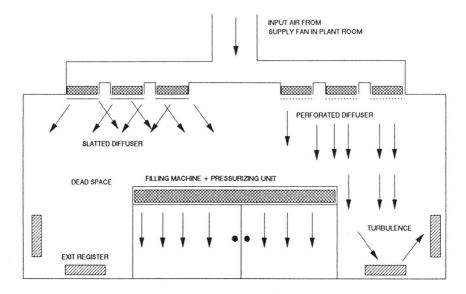

Fig. 8 Turbulent flow (conventional) clean room.

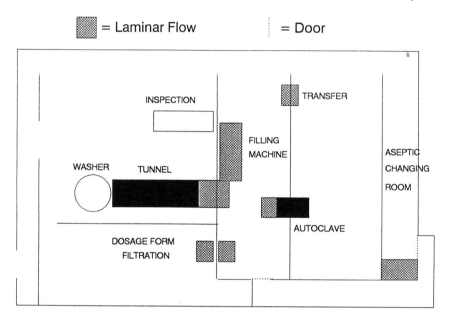

Fig. 9 Floor plan—aseptic vial filling line.

Figure 9 illustrates a liquid dosage form vial filling line with dedicated service areas. The flow of vials from empty to full follows a U-shaped track via a washing/LAF sterilizing/cooling tunnel positioned parallel to an inspection machine. The two arms of the U are connected by a localized laminar flow protected filling machine located in a Class 100 aseptic filling room.

In this facility there are two major gray areas, and the filling room lies between them. The dosage form is compounded and mixed in the same major gray area into which vials enter empty and leave filled but separated from these activities by a partition. Closures are processed through a double-ended rotary-drum washer/autoclave located in the second gray area on the other side of the filling room. The aseptic changing area and the laundry are located beside one another; both are protected by horizontal laminar flow.

In Fig. 10, two solid dosage form aseptic filling rooms share common gray areas. Once again the flow of vials from empty to full follows a U-shaped track, and again there are two major gray areas. Within each gray area the same personnel can service both lines with vials or closures.

There is no compounding or mixing in this process. The dosage form is received sterile from primary manufacture and is passed into the sterile area through a laminar flow protected interlocked transfer hatch. The dosage form containers are thoroughly decontaminated before being placed in the transfer

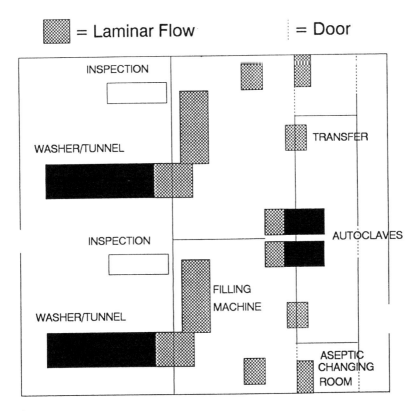

Fig. 10 Floor plan—twin vial filling lines.

hatch. Storage of these containers within the aseptic filling room is under local-ized laminar protection.

Figure 11 shows an aseptic manufacturing process in which several filling machines are located partially segregated in the same aseptic filling room. Each filling machine is separately provided with vials through dedicated washing/sterilizing/cooling tunnels. All filling machines are provided with sterile plugs via the same rotary drum washer/autoclave located in the second gray area on the other side of the filling room. Cross-flow of dosage forms and plugs complicates product control in such layouts. Additionally, the presence of sufficient staff in one filling room to operate all four filling machines introduces a significantly increased risk of microbiological contamination.

4. Clean Room Standards and Room Classification: Clean room technology is the most typical feature of aseptic manufacture. The major regulatory sources of guidance to appropriate technology and air standards for aseptic filling [2,3,4]

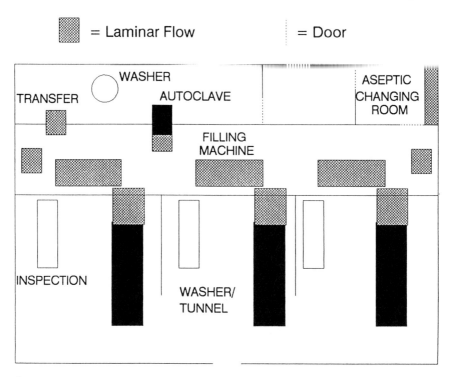

Fig. 11   Floor plan—multipurpose vial filling room.

lean heavily on two published *Clean Room Standards, Federal Standard 209* [5,6] and *British Standard 5295* for supportive details of how to evaluate the effectiveness of clean rooms. The *Clean Room Standards* classify clean rooms according to levels of physical particles of specified sizes present in air; importantly they describe how, where, and how often measurements must be made to permit the classification to be claimed. The concentration of physical particles in unit volume of air is regarded as a reliable index of the concentration of viable particles.

The most recent revisions of the two *Clean Room Standards* are *FS 209E* [22] in 1992 and *BS 5295.1989* [8] in 1989.

Federal Standard 209 has passed through five revisions, A, B, C, D and E. *FS 209A* was published in 1966. *FS 209B* was published in 1973 and was to all intents and purposes the basic reference document for air-borne contamination control throughout the world until 1988, when *FS 209D* was published. (*FS 209C* was a short-lived precursor to *FS 209D*.) The language of room classification has for many years been the language of the Federal Standard; Class 100, Class 10,000, etc., providing a clear graphic expression of the number of particles per unit volume (in this case per ft^3) of air within a classification and of the numerical relationships between classes. The most recent revision, *FS 209E* [22], published in 1992, has replaced this familiar classification with a new system of metric (SI) classifications and alternate nomenclatures. The new class limits are the metric equivalent (per m^3) of the previous class limits. The new names are derived from the logarithm to the base 10 of the metric class limits; Class 100 becomes Class M 3.5, Class 10,000 becomes Class M 5.5, etc. The nomenclature of previous revisions of *FS 209* is still permitted and will no doubt continue to be used for a good many years. The new nomenclature has little to commend it except that it can be decoded simply into metric class limits.

BS 5295 was first published in 1976; its room classification standards were strictly comparable to those of *FS 209B* except for approximations needed to convert imperial units *(FS 209B)* to metric units *(BS 5295)*.

The two *Clean Room Standards FS 209* and *BS 5295* are referenced in the regulatory documents governing aseptic filling. Table 1 compares the air classifications recommended or required for aseptic filling clean rooms in these pharmaceutical regulatory documents and references the particular *Standards* cited in support. Strictly speaking, the only options for room classification are the 1976 revision of *BS 5295* and the 1973 and 1988 revisions of *FS 209*.

In practical terms, these options can be extended to include the latest revisions of the *Clean Room Standards*. The EEC guidelines [4] for instance are (with subsequent revisions) keeping pace with the latest revision of *FS 209*. Although the limits of the classes are very much the same throughout these *Standards,* the type of testing and the amount of testing required to substantiate a claim to classification may differ significantly from one *Standard* to another. In particular, classification to *BS 5295.1989* requires far more testing than classification to any one of the other three *Standards*. Currently none of the major pharmaceutical regulatory documents require classification to *BS 5295.1989,* but it is possible that chauvinism and the "latest revision" concept will lead to this *Standard* being progressively adopted in European regulatory requirements.

Table 1 Clean Room Classes Recommended for Aseptic Filling (White Areas)

Pharmaceutical guidance document	Designation of class for aseptic manufacture	Referenced clean room standard class	Referenced clean room standard
"Orange Guide" [3]	Grade 1B	100	FS 209B
		1	BS 5295.1976
FDA *Guideline* [2]	No special designation	100	FS 209B
EEC *Guideline* [4]	Grade B	100	FS 209D

Classification of manufacturing environments in *Clean Room Standards* is based on numbers of physical particles of specified sizes present in unit volume of air. Particles of six size ranges (equal to or greater than 0.2 µm, 0.3 µm, 0.5 µm, 1 µm, 5 µm and 10 µm) are cited. Unit volume is described as per ft³ in the 1973 *Federal Standard,* per m³ in the *British Standard* and in the 1992 *Federal Standard.*   Classes are defined as numbers in the *Federal Standards* (Classes 100, 1,000, 10,000, and 100,000 in *FS 209B,* and M 3.5, M 5.5, and M 6.5 in *FS 209E*) and *BS 5295.1976* (Classes 1, 2 and 3); in *BS 5295.1989* classes are defined by letters of the alphabet (Classes E, F, G, H, J, and K). Table 2 compares the various classifications.

The traditional application of physical particulate standards to the pharmaceutical and medical devices industries has focussed on particle sizes equal to or greater than 0.5 µm and equal to or greater than 5 µm. Monitoring equipment has been specified to this end. Progressive revision of the *Clean Room Standards* has led to an increasing emphasis on smaller sized particles requiring more highly specified instrumentation for monitoring. *FS 209D* and *FS 209E* for instance now include class limits for particles of equal to and greater than 0.2 µm and 0.3 µm within Class 100 (Class M 3.5).

Considering the sizes of microorganisms and the sizes of the particles upon which air-borne microorganisms are likely to be carried (Fig. 12), it is very doubtful whether contamination from exceedingly small particles of less than 0.5 µm diameter are of sufficient relevance to the pharmaceutical industry to

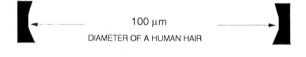

100 µm
DIAMETER OF A HUMAN HAIR

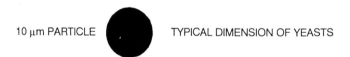

10 µm PARTICLE   TYPICAL DIMENSION OF YEASTS

0.5 µm PARTICLE ● TYPICAL DIMENSION OF BACTERIA

Fig. 12 Relative sizes of particles.

Table 2 Comparison of Particle Count Requirements in Clean Room Standards Applicable to Aseptic Filling (FS 209 Class 100 [M 3.5], BS 5295.1976 Class 1, BS 5295.1989 Classes E and F)

	Validation				Routine monitoring			
	BS 5295		FS 209		BS 5295		FS 209	
	1976	1989	B(1973)	E(1992)	1976	1989	B(1973)	E(1992)
Minimum number of locations per room	3	NS	2	2	3	NS	AS	AS
Recommended floor area per sample location	20–25 m²	10 m²	Area in ft² divided by 10	Area in ft² divided by 10	20–25 m²	10 m²	AS	AS
Locations to be sampled	Close to walls work stations & where control is important	Equal subareas	Uniformly spaced	Uniformly spaced	Close to walls work stations & where control is important	Equal subareas	AS or where cleanliness is critical, or high counts in validation	AS
Replication at each location	NS	×5	NS	NS	NS	×5	NS	NS
Recommended frequency	NS	At least once per year and after closure exceeds 7 d	Initial & periodic	AS	Daily	Weekly	AS	AS

NS = not specified; AS = as otherwise specified.

merit wholesale replacement of instrumentation unless the revised *Standards* are imposed by regulatory pressure over-enthusiasm for the "latest revision" concept could too easily lead to unwarranted emphasis on very small particles and over-emphasis on air-borne contamination to the detriment of the greater risk of surface-to-surface contamination from personnel working in aseptic facilities.

The FDA's *Guideline on Sterile Drug Products Produced by Aseptic Processing* [2] requires Class 100 conditions of *FS 209B* for aseptic filling rooms; the *Orange Guide* [3] asks for Class 1 of *BS 5295.1973* or Class 100 of *FS* 209B. Classification of clean rooms to these *Standards* does not require measurement of particles smaller than 0.5 µm. The EEC Guideline [4] however refers to *FS 209D*, which additionally requires measurement of particles equal to or greater than 0.2 µm and 0.3 µm. There is no evidence of regulatory insistence on measurement of these particle sizes. It is probably reasonable to assume that any future revision of the FDA *Guideline* is likely to follow suit and change its *Standard from FS 209B* to *FS 209E*, which contains the same provisions. It is to be hoped that any such revision should specifically exclude the measurement and monitoring of particles smaller than 0.5 µm.

 a. Sampling Requirements for Clean Room Classification. In the *Clean Room Standards,* sampling is considered for two circumstances, for validation (termed certification in the *Standards*) and for routine monitoring. Further distinctions may be made on the basis of the operational condition of the clean room when samples are taken. *The Standards* of the 1970s are quite explicit. *FS 209B* states that "counts are to be taken during work activity periods." *BS 5295.1976* requires validation to be done in the unmanned state and routine monitoring in the manned state.

The *Standards* of the 1980s and 1990s allow classification to be claimed for "as built," manned or unmanned conditions (*BS 5295.1989*), or "as built," "at rest," operational, or "as otherwise specified" (*FS 209D* and *FS 209E*). This increased scope in the *Clean Room Standards* is not helpful to interpreting the pharmaceutical regulatory literature that predates their publication. The documents offering guidance on aseptic filling make sparse reference to the operational state under which clean room classification should be claimed.

Some types of aseptic filling are not suited to particle counting while operational at all; for instance, solid dosage forms generate particles from the product itself; classification to *FS 209B* has always been interpreted freely to accommodate this. Other types of manufacturing equipment are particle generators when in operation. It is partly to prevent contamination from these sources that localized protection is so widely advocated for pharmaceutical manufacture. A footnote to *FS 209D* states that the "as otherwise specified" condition should refer to the degree of control specified by the user or contracting agency. This may be regarded fairly as an invitation to specialized industries such as aseptic pharmaceutical manufacturers to derive their own requirements for clean room classification while remaining within the overall coverage of the *Clean Room Standard.* Normal practice is for classification to be done in the unmanned nonoperational condition.

Classification and monitoring to the *Clean Room Standards* requires that particular numbers of samples of air be taken per unit floor area, that samples be taken in specified locations, and that samples be taken at appropriate frequencies. Table 2 summarizes these requirements. It is evident that the evolution of the US standard from *FS 209B* to *FS 209E*, both for validation and for routine monitoring, is toward the "as otherwise specified" condition, which bounces the onus for decision-making back to the user and his "customer." This is not the case for the *British Standard.* To validate a clean room, the *British Standard BS 5295.1989* asks for more locations and more replicate testing at each location than *BS 5295.1976* or either revision of the U.S. standard.

In *BS 5295.1989*, conditions for routine particle monitoring are no less demanding than those specified for validation. The frequency for routine monitoring is weekly versus monthly for *FS 209D*.

This means that the amount of testing required to claim compliance with *BS 5295.1989* is far higher than the amount of testing required to claim compliance for the same clean room with any other standard.

Figure 13 illustrates sampling locations to *BS 5295.1989* and *FS 209D* (and *FS 209E*) for an aseptic filling clean room approximately 7.3 by 11.3 m (82

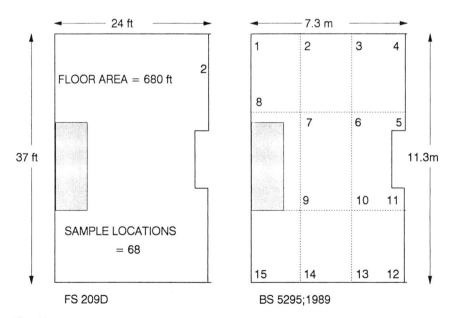

Fig. 13 Sampling locations for compliance with Clean Room Standards BS 5295.1989 and FS 209D.

m^2). *FS 209D* requires the largest number of locations, 68; *BS 5295.1989* specifies 15 locations, but with 5 replications this amounts to about the same number
of samples, 70, as *FS 209D*. It is only when it comes to routine monitoring that
the full impact of selecting compliance with one or other of the two 1980s standards becomes apparent. *FS 209D* asks for monthly monitoring and allows the
user and "customer" to agree on the number and location of monitoring points.
FS 209E allows the frequency of routine monitoring to be "as specified." *BS
5295.1989* demands a weekly repetition of the particle counting exercise done
for validation.

Clearly there are issues here that the pharmaceutical industry needs to
address. Particles of the smaller sizes specified for measurement in the *Clean
Room Standards* are not of direct concern to particulate contamination issues
facing manufacturers of sterile pharmaceuticals. Furthermore, it is the quality of
clean room technology that is the factor of greatest importance to the pharmaceutical industry, of which the attainment of clean room classification is merely
an indirect index. In these circumstances a major increase in the amount of
testing required to claim compliance with a particular classification offers no
benefit to the industry, and may indeed unnecessarily increase testing costs,
downtime. etc.

b. Tests on Filters. The two most important specifications for HEPA
filters are the specified efficiency of the filter media and the specified integrity
of the filter as installed (the leak test).

Table 3 compares the minimum filter efficiencies cited in the guidance
documents on aseptic manufacturing and in the *Clean Room Standards*. It is
curious that the specification for filter efficiency in the *"Orange Guide"* is
tighter than the specifications given in the two *Clean Room Standards* it refer-

Table 3 Comparison of Minimum Filter Efficiencies Referenced in
Guides to Aseptic Pharmaceutical Manufacture and Clean Room Standards

Document	Minimum filter efficiency
"Orange Guide" [3]	99.997%[a]
FDA *Guideline* [2]	99.97%[b]
EEC *Guideline* [4]	Appropriate
FS 209B [5] - Class 100	99.97%[b]
FS 209D [6] - Class 100	NS
FS 209E [22] - Class M 3.5	NS
BS 5295 - 1976 [7] - Class 1	99.995%[a]
BS 5295 - 1989 [8] - Classes E and F	95%

NS = Not specified; [a]Tested according to BS 3928; [b]Tested according to MIL-F-51065.

Table 4 Comparison of Maximum Acceptable Percentage Recoveries of Upstream Challenge Particles in Filter Installation Integrity Tests Referenced in Guides to Aseptic Pharmaceutical Manufacture and Clean Room Standards

Document	Maximum % recovery
"Orange Guide" [3]	NS
FDA *Guideline* [2]	0.01
EEC *Guideline* [4]	NS
FS 209B [5] - Class 100	0.01
FS 209D [6] - Class 100	NS
FS 209E [22] - Class M 3.5	NS
BS 5295 - 1976 [7] - Class 1	0.01
BS 5295 - 1989 [8] - Classes E and F	0.001

NS = Not specified.

ences *(FS 209B* and *BS 5295.1976).* The FDA Guideline does not require such a high standard of filter efficiency (99.97% versus 99.997%).

Table 4 compares the maximum acceptable percentage of the upstream concentration of a challenge population of particles that can be recovered downstream of the filter. *BS 5295.1989* is exceptional in requiring no more than 0.001% for Classes E and F (nearest classification to Class 100 of the Federal standards); the nearest specification in the other documents is 0.01%. The implications of *BS 5295.1989* to test methodology are significant; instrumentation that is sufficiently sensitive to meet other standards is not necessarily of sufficient sensitivity to meet BS *5295.1989.*

Overall, the standards being adopted worldwide for classification of aseptic pharmaceutical filling rooms are those of *FS 209.* This is because of the practical flexibility of this standard. The *British Standard* has diverged from strict equivalence with its introduction of levels of testing activity that may be more appropriate to the electronics industry. The availability of *Clean Room Standards* has been important to the development and responsible control of aseptic manufacture over the past 30 years or so. In the immediate future it remains to resolve how the same *Standards* can address the needs of the electronics industry and pharmaceutical industries without compromising one or the other.

C. Specific Aseptic Systems

Vial filling has been used to exemplify typical aseptic filling processes. It is, of course, an important application, but there are other applications peculiar to specific product contact containers that merit separate treatment. These include glass ampoules, form-fill-sealed plastic ampoules, and lyophilization.

1   Glass Ampoules: Glass ampoules are narrow necked single piece containers sealed by fusion of the glass. Most ampoules are pull-sealed. The neck of the ampoule is heated by high temperature burners directed at an area close to the tip but leaving enough of the tip to be held firmly in mechanical jaws. The ampoule is rotated in the flame to ensure even heating. When the glass has softened sufficiently, the tip is pulled rapidly away from the body of the ampoule. The ampoule continues to rotate, twisting closed any unfused capillary.

Alternatively, ampoules may be tip-sealed. The ampoule is rotated while being heated in the burners or it is heated by means of a pair of burners, one on each side of the ampoule. Sealing is by fusion of a bead of glass at the tip of the ampoule.

The absence of separate closures dictates different aseptic systems to vial filling, for instance, there are no closures to wash and sterilize. The ampoules themselves require to be treated in a very similar way to vials with respect to washing and sterilization prior to filling. Two types of ampoule may be purchased for aseptic filling; they may be purchased as "open" or purchased as "sealed by the supplier." It is necessary to wash open ampoules in gray areas before dry heat sterilization and filling. "Sealed by the supplier" ampoules are not necessarily washed if there is sufficient confidence in the supplier's processes, but they must be cut open before sterilization and filling. One of the major product and patient related problems associated with ampoules is glass spicules, which can allegedly be causative agents of pulmonary embolism. These spicules may arise during manufacture from opening "sealed by the supplier" ampoules or at point of use from opening by the user. Positive pressures within ampoules may reduce the amount of particulate contamination arising from opening.

2. Form-Fill-Seal: The form-fill-seal process is one in which the primary container for the dosage form is formed from a thermoplastic, aseptically filled, and then sealed in one integrated system. The technology has spread from the food industry into sterile pharmaceuticals via products for respiratory therapy (nebules for nebulizers), which are required to be single dose but which are not required to be sterile. Many of the fundamental materials concerns regarding permeation, leaching, chemical reactivity, toxicity, and extractives were resolved for these products. Pharmaceutically inert formulations of polyethylene, polypropylene, and various copolymers and polyallomers are commercially available and suitable for pharmaceutical form-fill-seal applications.

At the heart of the process is the blow-molding machine. This technology is not unique to aseptic processing. In the machine, molten plastic is extruded under high temperatures (around 200°C) and pressures (350 bar) as a hollow

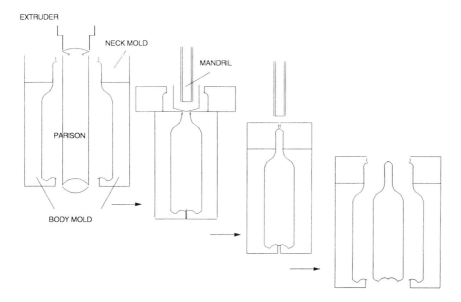

Fig. 14 Blow-fill-seal process.

tube (Fig. 14). The extruded material (the "parison"), while still molten, is then fed between two mirror image halves of a die in the shape of the container to be formed. The two halves of the die close around the parison and seal it at its base. A mandril is inserted automatically into the neck of the partially formed container to blow high-pressure air into the mold thus forming the body of the container.

The process becomes somewhat more elaborate for aseptic filling [9]. In order to combine the processes of molding and filling, the mandril comprises two concentric tubes. The outer tube delivers the air to form the container—for aseptic filling the air must of course be filter sterilized—the inner tube delivers the aseptically filtered dosage form.

The final stage of the system is the removal of the mandril followed immediately by closure of the two halves of the part of the mold which forms the neck of the container. The whole process takes no longer than 10 to 15 s, and several containers can be formed, filled, and sealed in parallel molds within this time frame.

This type of technology has given rise to some considerable amount of debate within the pharmaceutical industry and the regulatory bodies. Concerns about the cleanliness of the machinery and contamination of the polymer granules have been largely resolved; so also have issues surrounding the quality of the services (cooling water, hydraulic fluids, etc.). The main area of contention has been the necessity or lack of necessity for these machines to be operated in high-quality clean rooms.

The whole operation of forming a sterile container, filling it, and sealing it, is conducted within one machine. The filling zone for aseptic filling is afforded localized filtered air protection. There is no intervention from personnel until after the filled presentation is sealed and automatically moved away from the point of fill. What need therefore for location within a Class 100 clean room, or for protection by the "double barrier" principle? Support for this argument has come mainly from media fill studies conducted with machines located in Class 10,000 areas [10]. Accumulation of uncontaminated individual trials, each of several units of thousands of items to total numbers of several tens and even hundreds of thousands of items has been used to claim equivalence between form-fill-seal in Class 10,000 clean rooms with conventional "double-barrier" aseptic fill in Class 100 clean rooms.

While form-fill-seal aseptic processing is undoubtably very effective and safe, the counter argument has it that better assurance of sterility would be obtained by giving this type of machinery the same degree of protection given to conventional aseptic filling machines. Supporters of this view point out that media fill results are a grossly insensitive system of measuring the actual levels of sterility assurance obtained from aseptic processing (see below), and that the accumulation of results from separate trials or universes is statistically invalid. Less theoretically, a recent practical investigation of form-fill-seal technology in an artificially contaminated environment [11] has indicated that the level of sterility assurance obtained with specific form-fill-seal technologies is clearly a function (albeit a complex function) of the microbiological quality of the environment in which the machinery is housed.

3. Lyophilization (Freeze Drying): Lyophilization is most frequently used for heat-labile dosage forms that are unstable in aqueous formulation. The principle of lyophilization can be seen by reference to the phase equilibrium diagram for water (Fig. 15). Water at atmospheric pressure and ambient temperatures is stable in its liquid phase; at 100°C the liquid phase attains an equilibrium with its vapor phase. Above 100°C water is stable in its vapor phase. At atmospheric pressures and 0°C the solid (ice) and liquid phases of water are in equilibrium with each other. At vacuum pressures a temperature (the eutectic point) can be reached where the three phases, solid, liquid, and vapor are all in equilibrium with each other. At even lower temperatures and pressures the solid phase comes into equilibrium with the liquid phase. The significance of this is that an aqueous solution can be concentrated by "evaporation" (sublimation) at low pressures without any necessity for significant heat input.

Figure 16 is a schematic representation of a lyophilizer. The most important features are the chamber, the condensor, which is separated from the chamber but attached by vapor lines, and the vacuum pumps. Within the chamber

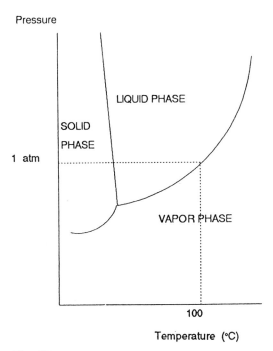

Fig. 15 Phase diagram for water.

there are four shelves, which can be refrigerated or heated according to the needs of the process. The chamber can be evacuated by a twin pump setup and is provided with air, nitrogen, and steam lines.

In essence the process comprises six stages:

(a) Filling. The dosage form is compounded in concentrated aqueous formulation, sterilized by filtration through 0.22 μm membranes, and aseptically filled into unsealed vials. Protection from gross contamination is often afforded by the final closures being loosely inserted in the vial necks.

(b) Freezing. This is done with the vials loaded into trays designed to fit into the refrigerated shelves in the chamber of the lyophilizer. Freezing may take several hours.

(c) Evacuation. The chamber of the lyophilizer is evacuated to low pressure.

(d) Sublimation. Water vapor subliming from the frozen dosage form is condensed on heat exchanger surfaces held at or around −50°C within the lyophilizer.

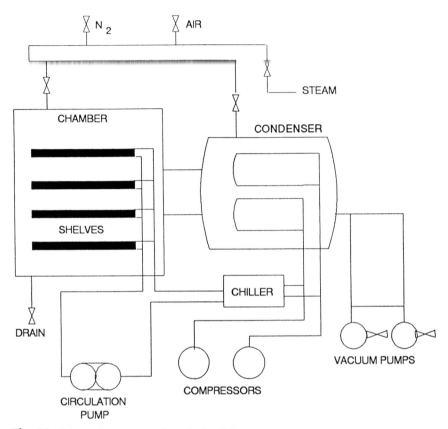

Fig. 16 Schematic representation of a lyophilizer.

(e) Heating. The rate of sublimation increases with increasing temperature at temperatures below the eutectic temperature. Controlled heating is a normal feature of commercial lyophilization. Care must be exercised to avoid heat-induced product degradation. The complete cycle to less than 1% moisture may take as long as 24 h, depending on the surface-to-volume ratio of the dosage form.

(f) Sealing. At the end of the process, sterile air, nitrogen, or other appropriate inert gas is bled into the chamber and the closures are forced home by rams or by movement of one shelf against the one above.

Lyophilization has several stages and subprocesses beyond aseptic vial filling that increase the potential for contamination and introduce additional requirements for sterilization. First, vials for lyophilization are usually trayed and loaded into and unloaded out of the chamber manually. This in itself creates a greater risk of product contamination than less labor-intensive processes. Second, trays require sterilization, and so too does the lyophilizer itself. Lyophilizers are usually sterilized by ethylene oxide or by high-temperature steam (as represented in Fig. 16); processes of sterilization have to be addressed for thermal and biological effectiveness in the same way as sterilizing autoclaves.

III. STERILITY ASSURANCE FROM ASEPTIC FILLING

It is not possible to measure levels of sterility assurance (SALs) obtained with commercial systems of achieving sterility. The expected assurance of sterility is too high to be measurable by techniques that rely on detection of nonsterility in sampled items. With processes that involve microbiological inactivation, measurements of subprocess inactivation can be extrapolated to estimate process SALs. This not possible for aseptic filling.

The "spirit" of aseptic manufacture is that if every precautionary measure is operating correctly there should be very little risk of product contamination. Furthermore, a product item that becomes microbiologically contaminated during manufacture is not necessarily a nonsterile item when it comes to be used. Microorganisms must survive as well as contaminate products for the products to contain viable microorganisms (i.e., to be nonsterile) at the significant time of the product being administered to the patient. Many pharmaceutically active agents are intrinsically antimicrobial, and many dosage forms are formulated to be antimicrobial. Derivation of SALs for aseptically filled products, comparable to those which can be derived for terminally sterilized products, is therefore at best a very complex exercise, at worst a futile one.

The FDA has indicated [12] that it expects the same SALs for all supposedly sterile products irrespective of the method of manufacture, and that acceptable SALs should be no worse than 10^{-6}. Practically, aseptic manufacturing systems are validated (see below) by establishing that each individual process is doing what it is supposed to do, and then integrating these systems by reference to a biological test, the media fill or simulation trial. Media fills determine an upper limit for SALs based on probabilities of contamination that may result from particular filling processes. Media fills provide no data on survival of microorganisms in products; they do not therefore constitute a measure of product SALs.

In its simplest form, the simulation trial substitutes microbial growth media for actual product and scores containers for growth or absence of growth after incubation. The media fill is a measure of potential contamination. It is to be assumed that properly chosen and properly controlled microbiological media will encourage rather than inhibit the survival of contaminants. This is quite the opposite effect on microorganisms to that which most pharmaceutical dosage forms are formulated to have.

The acceptable standard to be achieved in simulation trials is for there to be no more than 1 contaminated item in 1000 items. This limit, which has been established on the basis of the probability of false positives arising in microbiological transfers being in the region of 10^{-3}, is frequently interpreted to mean that SALs actually achieved for aseptically manufactured products are no better than 10^{-3}. This interpretation is not correct. Media fill results apply to the aseptic system, not to the products being passed through the system. SALs in products are a function of the probability of items becoming contaminated and of those contaminants surviving. The media fill provides only the first factor in such an equation, such that even in the unlikely event of all contaminants surviving (probability of survival equal to 1) the product SAL would be no worse than 10^{-3}.

In 1981 Whyte [13] proposed a model to describe the potential probability of microbiological contamination of the contents of containers originating from the air in the environment of aseptic filling rooms. The model incorporated three additive effects:

(a) The first factor in this model assumed that the rate at which particles settle out of the air onto horizontal surfaces is largely dependent upon the size of the particles. Assuming Stoke's law and an average contaminated particle diameter of 12 µm, the number of particles deposited from air into an open container can be described by the expression

Number of particles deposited $= 0.0032 \cdot d^2 \cdot C \cdot A_n \cdot t$

where d = equivalent particle diameter (µm), C = airborne particle concentration per cm^3, A_n = area of the opening of the neck of the container, and t = time the container is open (s).

(b) Another mechanism which he considered was that contamination could arise from particles from an airstream being thrown into the open neck of the container. Whyte presumed that the greatest risk of contamination of the contents of a container by impaction from this source would be from air flowing parallel to the neck of the container. He quantified this risk as

Number of particles impacted $= C \cdot A_n \cdot V \cdot E \cdot t$

where V = air velocity parallel to the neck of the container (cm/s), and

$$E = 3.27 \times \frac{10^{-6} \cdot V \cdot d^2}{l}$$

where l = diameter of the neck of the container (cm).

(c) Third, he assumed that the particle concentration within a container left open will eventually equilibrate to the same particle concentration as the room air. The contribution to contamination from this source is

Number of particles from inside the container $= C \cdot V_b$

where V_b = volume of container in cm^3. This is of course a very conservative clause in Whyte's model, because good filling room practice will not allow containers to remain open long enough to equilibrate with the environment.

Allowing that there are a substantial number of unconfirmed assumptions supporting Whyte's model, it is likely that its prediction of the probability of contamination from air-borne sources is not too far wrong. Consider therefore that the probability of contamination arising in 20 mL vials remaining open for as long as 30 s under Class 100 conditions (equivalent according to Whyte to 3.5×10^{-6} air-borne viable particles per cm^3) can be calculated to be in the region of 10^{-5}.

Calculations and models of this type confirm that actual SALs obtained for aseptically filled products are far better than would be suggested from simulation trial results alone, and in fact far closer to the generally accepted SAL of 10^{-6} applied to terminally sterilized products.

These models also suggest that one or more subsystems within the overall systems of aseptic control may fail, yet simulation trials may remain satisfactory. Although the simulation trial is a valuable tool toward revealing systems failure, it is in fact an insensitive one; therefore not too much credence should be given to long sequences of satisfactory results. Independent systems may be failing and causing extreme fluctuations in actual SALs without these being detected within the limits of sensitivity of the simulation trials.

SALs obtained from aseptic filling processes have been modelled from theoretical considerations and are probably as good as 10^{-5} or better. The simulation trial is an insensitive tool that cannot within reasonable experimental dimensions confirm SALs better than 10^{-3}. It is not to be assumed that an aseptic filling process is under control merely because a series of satisfactory simulation trials with less than one contaminated item in one thousand have been obtained. Adequate assurance of sterility can only be obtained by ensuring that all possible precautions against contamination are in place and that each one is performing in the manner intended.

IV. VALIDATION AND CONTROL OF ASEPTIC MANUFACTURE

Aseptic manufacture is one of the most technically demanding operations in the pharmaceutical industry. To provide adequate assurance of sterility it is necessary to demonstrate that every critical mechanism and protective system consistently fulfills its intended purpose. A degree of overkill cannot be built in to a passive target couched in absolute terms—total protection from contamination.

Thorough and well founded validation is therefore imperative. Routine monitoring is merely an extension of validation, and ongoing control comprises the systems of response not only to excursions beyond predetermined monitoring tolerances but also to potentially deleterious trends that may become evident within those tolerances.

A. Validation

The first stage in the design of a validation system for an aseptic manufacturing operation is a detailed analysis of the process into its unit operations. In this way it is possible to identify those systems and subsystems that have an effect on the potential microbiological quality of the product. This exercise must include those systems intended to reduce contamination by washing, by disinfection, or by sterilization, which have independent validation requirements, as well as the specific aseptic systems intended to prevent contamination of the dosage form and product contact components. The validation program should address and document each of these systems. Consistency over time should be addressed through periodic revalidation. By and large, routine monitoring only addresses those systems that can be monitored without causing major disruption to manufacture. Many aseptic control systems do not fall into this category and must therefore be revisited for validation purposes at intervals well within their expected shelf life.

The supposed biological integration of the individual effectivenesses of these systems is by completion of satisfactory media filling trials. This does not mean that filling trial should be considered as a substitute to validation of each individual process that may impact upon product contamination. As stated above, filling trials are in fact a poor measure of the degree of protection from contamination that is expected and indeed obtainable from aseptic manufacture. Regardless of this, the filling trial is recognized to be the only approach to integration currently available. Current regulatory thinking is that it is an absolute necessity.

The following pages identify the principal individual aseptic systems that must be validated and appropriate standards to be met.

1. Instrumentation: All instrumentation, measuring devices, and alarm systems installed on equipment and in facilities intended for aseptic manufacture should be ascertained to read or react over appropriately specified ranges. Complex equipment should be designed to allow access to measuring devices for calibration or removal for calibration. Calibration of the signal from the measuring device is not sufficient without the measuring device itself being checked.

A properly controlled system of calibration is necessary. Calibration is defined [15] as the comparison of a measurement system or device of unknown accuracy to another measurement system or device of known accuracy. The purpose of calibration is to correlate the two devices, or eliminate by adjustment any variation from the required performance limits of the unverified measurement system or device. In other words, it determines the accuracy of an item of measuring equipment. Any adjustment made to a measuring device since last calibrated should be recorded and reviewed; measuring devices that lose their calibration easily should be calibrated at a frequency designed to avoid significant consequences arising from loss of accuracy.

Calibration should be traceable to national or international standards through an unbroken chain of comparisons. For instrumentation affecting sterility control in aseptic manufacturing facilities this usually involves comparison of values measured with the item of equipment under test, say a particle counter or a pressure differential gauge, with values measured with a standardized device. In many cases this may mean the use of external contract calibration services, with all that this implies in relation to assuring that the contractor's calibration control systems are themselves under good control.

An integral aspect of instrumentation validation is that not only should all instruments be calibrated when first installed but that they should also be recalibrated at fixed or variable intervals. These intervals should be established on some sensible basis that is intended to ensure that instrumentation will meet its required accuracy specifications throughout all periods of usage.

This may mean calibration at predetermined intervals of time or predetermined intervals based on utilization. The requirement for recalibration may well help define a schedule for routine preventative maintenance.

Complete records of all calibrations should be maintained. This must include unique identification of each item of instrumentation, its location within the aseptic manufacturing facility, and its calibration history and evidence of its traceability to recognized standards.

All instrumentation within aseptic manufacturing facilities should be identified during validation, and the potential of each instrument for causing deleterious effects to sterility should be independently evaluated. All instruments should be calibrated and scheduled for routine recalibration and for routine preventative maintenance. A system should be set up to ensure that any failure to meet these predetermined schedules is flagged to Quality Assurance to evaluate the effect on sterility.

2. *Facilities*: The fabric and fittings of aseptic manufacturing facilities should be reviewed during validation and when the facility is revalidated. Even with new facilities it is possible for builders or contractors to have modified the intended specifications. With older facilities it is not unknown to find unaccept-

able changes made to fabric or fittings as a result of modification or maintenance activities. Services in particular should be ascertained to being provided from outside aseptic filling rooms, new electrical fittings should be flush to walls or ceilings, and any incidental damage to walls, floors, or ceilings should have been made good.

The major system of contamination control is the air handling system. The various exercises that make up the validation of air handling systems are common to both white and gray areas. It is only the standards that differ (Table 5).

Table 5 Comparison of Air Standards for White and Gray Areas

	Number of particles per m³ (Approximate figures per ft³ in parentheses) of size equal to or greater than . . .				
White area standards	0.3 μm	0.5 μm	1 μm	5 μm	10 μm
BS5295 : 1976 Class 1 [7]	—	3,000	—	0	0
BS5295 : 1989 Class E [8]	10,000 (300)	3,500 (100)	—	0	0
BS5295 : 1989 Class F [8]	—	3,500 (100)	—	0	0
FS209B : Class 100 [5]	—	3,500 (100)	—	0	0
FS209D : Class 100 [6]	10,500 (300)	3,500 (100)	—	—	—
Gray Area Standards					
BS5295 : 1976 Class 2 [7]	—	300,000 (10,000)	—	2,000	30
BS5295 : 1989 Class J [8]	—	350,000 (10,000)	—	2,000 (70)	0
BS5295 : 1989 Class K [8]	—	3,500,000 (100,000)	—	20,000 (700)	450 (150)
FS209B : Class 10,000 [5]	—	350,000 (10,000)	—	2,500 (65)	—
FS209B : Class 100,000 [5]	—	3,500,000 (100,000)	—	25,000 (700)	—
FS209D : Class 10,000 [6]	—	350,000 (10,000)	—	2,500 (70)	—
SF209D : Class 100,000 [6]	—	3,500,000 (100,000)	—	25,000 (700)	—

a. Validation of HEPA Filters. There are two important specifications for filters intended to produce high-quality, microorganism-free air. These are the specified efficiency of the filter medium and the specified integrity of the filter as installed (the leak test or DOP test).

The former is specified by the manufacturer, determined according to the penetration of particles of sodium chloride with mass median diameters of 0.6 μm and need not be verified as part of the validation program.

The leak test or DOP test (named after dioctyl phthallate, the original but now rarely used oil source) is an *in situ* test to verify that filters do not leak on installation. The leak test is not a second efficiency test. It is intended to disclose leaks around the frames and damage to the filter medium. An aerosol of oil particles with mass median diameter of 0.3 μm is used to challenge the filter; detection is by aerosol photometry on the downstream side. Standards of integrity are specified as maximum permissable percentages of the upstream concentration of particles that can be recovered downstream of the filter.

b. Validation of Air Circulation. There are three factors relating to air circulation that are important to the validation of aseptic manufacture. These are air velocities, airflow patterns, and air exchange rates.

Achievement of satisfactory air velocities is imperative to laminar flow installations. The laminarity and the sweeping effects that are essential to their effective operation are functions of air velocity. The standard within the pharmaceutical industry is an average velocity of 90 ft/min with a plus or minus 20% tolerance.

The problem is where to measure the velocity? The options are close to the filter face, in the working area, or at the extremities of the protected area (air exiting from, say, the curtains of a vertical laminar flow canopy). The resolution of where to measure may not be easy. For instance the filter face of a large vertical flow canopy shrouding a filling machine may be more than 1 m above the filling zone. By and large the pharmaceutical industry has chosen to measure air velocity close to the filter face.

The basis of modern aseptic manufacturing technology is airflow protection. Airflow patterns determine the effectiveness of airflow protection. Where does the air from input registers or from laminar flow installations go? Is it sweeping over the areas that require protection? Is the airflow causing eddies and dead space? None of this can be accurately predicted. There are no standards to be met. This is purely a qualititative exercise that must be done empirically. The method is to use smoke pencils or to use a smoke generator and observation. None of this work can be done with an area sterile and operational. Records for referral and inspection are best maintained on film or video. Video cameras intended for underwater use can be decontaminated using disinfectants to minimize the potential for carrying microorganisms into clean areas.

The microbial and particulate quality of aseptic filling rooms is maintained by dilution as well as filtration. The rate of exchange of room air is important to the contribution made by dilution. Room air should be changed at least 20 times per hour. Around 90% of the air should be recycled through the filters. There should also be a satisfactory pressure differential (minimum 0.05 inches WG or 15 pascals) between clean rooms and adjacent less protected areas.

c. Room Classification. Classification of aseptic filling rooms and gray areas to clean room standards is an integral part of validation. The key technology is the measurement of concentrations of nonviable particles per unit volume of air. Classification has been addressed in some detail above.

In some instances the terminology of room classification may be used where it is neither specifically necessary nor specifically correct. The FDA *Guideline* [2] refers to a "per-cubic-foot particle count of no more than 100 in a size range of 0.5 μm and larger (Class 100) when measured not more than one foot away from the worksite and upstream of the air flow." The sampling requirements of the *Clean Room Standards* may be omitted when superfluous to the purposes of aseptic manufacture.

White areas (Class 100 clean rooms) should clean up to their classification within 20 min of starting up air handling systems unless there is some major particle generator present in the room or leaks in the ducting.

d. Microbiological Characteristics. All of the microbiological characteristics of aseptic manufacturing facilities described below under Routine Monitoring (Section IV.B) should also be completed during validation as a base line measurement of how things are when all systems are known to be operating in their intended manner.

3. Aseptic Filling Room Garments: Operators and their garments are potentially the most significant source of contamination of aseptic filling rooms. It should be ascertained that garments for use in aseptic filling rooms are made from materials that shed virtually no fibers or particulate matter and that they should retain microbial particles shed from the body. Fabric edges should be sealed and seams should be all enveloping. Validation records should include manufacturer's information on the barrier characteristics of the garment fabric, i.e., air permeability, pore size, and particle removal.

Garments should be laundered (or cleaned) and sterilized in an effective manner. Validation of the laundering process should demonstrate that both laundered and unlaundered garments are contaminated by no more than 5,000 particles of length greater than 0.5 μm and no more than 25 fibers (particles longer than 100 μm with a length-to-width ratio exceeding 10:1) according to ASTM F 51/68 [15].

Radiation is suitable for sterilizing aseptic area garments, with three provisos. First, plastic studs and zips should be avoided to prevent embrittlement creating sources of particles and loss of integrity. Second, radiation may accelerate the fading of some colored garments. This could be helpful to controlling the number of sterilization cycles through which the garments can be passed but is probably not the best way of doing this. Third, irradiated garments may carry an aroma of ozone to which some personnel may be sensitive. Types of steam sterilization cycle used to sterilize gowns and scrub suits in hospitals are unlikely to meet the same criteria for sterilization validation applied in the pharmaceutical industry. Validatable cycles may require very long poststerilization drying to guarantee against dampness.

4. Disinfectants and Cleaning Processes: Disinfectants are an integral part of cleaning processes for aseptic manufacture. They are usually purchased as concentrated stock solutions; for use they should be diluted in water of *Purified Water* or *Water for Injection* quality. They should be filtered into white areas, usually, because of their viscosity, through 0.45 μm sterilizing filters. Each diluted batch should be allocated a shelf-life, and different disinfectants should be used in documented rotation.

Validation of disinfectants should be concentrated on two aspects of their potential to create problems in aseptic manufacture. First, they may themselves be sources of microbiological contamination; second, they may not be effective against microbial contaminants.

Samples of disinfectants should be taken as close to their point of use as possible and examined for microbiological contamination by passage through 0.22 μm membrane filters. Great care must be taken to flush the membranes to ensure removal of any residual traces of disinfectant before they are placed in or on microbiological recovery media.

The effectiveness of disinfectants should also be evaluated. The approach to this is not as simple as it might seem. Very obviously, the simplest method is chemical analysis of the active ingredient. However, it is usual to find that this is supplemented by some form of microbiological data. The principles of microbiological testing of disinfectants go back to the Rideal-Walker method of 1903 and probably earlier. Even with this long history, disinfectant testing is not free, nor ever has been free, from criticism and controversy.

Whereas the real test of a disinfectant is in its practical application, the responsibility for evaluation lies in the laboratory. The resistance of microorganisms to disinfectants may vary widely, influenced by the presence of organic materials, the wetting capability of the surface being disinfected, the temperature at the time of application, and species-to-species, strain-to-strain, and phase-of-growth characteristics of target microorganisms. Laboratory tests attempt to control these factors within tighter limits than would ever be encountered in practice.

The basic concept is to compare the effectiveness of the proposed disinfectant with that of phenol by reference to a standard microorganism. The Association of Official Analytical Chemists is probably the best source of detailed state-of-the-art methodology. For validation of disinfectants for purposes of aseptic manufacture, the relevance of the test may be improved by including microorganisms representative of local contamination in the test.

5. *Liquids and Lubricants*: All automated filling equipment must require periodic lubrication. Wherever possible, lubricants should be sterilized prior to being brought into aseptic filling rooms, but in practice this is not always compatible with lubricating characteristics. Only sterilized lubricants should be used for any pieces of equipment that come into direct contact with the dosage form or product contact containers; for other applications within aseptic filling rooms, lubricants containing bactericides should only be used. These should be evaluated against reasonable standards of microbiological contamination (for instance, no more than one colony-forming unit per mL or gram).

6. *Media Filling Trials*: Media fills are intended to simulate the risk of contamination that may arise from the aseptic assembly of sterile product elements by substitution of a sterilized placebo for the dosage form. The placebo should be chosen to be of similar flow/filling performance characteristics to the sterilized dosage form to mimic accurately the normal conditions of the production process.

For aqueous liquid products the placebo most commonly used is a liquid microbiological growth medium (broth). For solid dosage form, placebos such as lactose, mannitol, and polyethylene glycol may be filled and microbiological growth medium added afterwards.

a. Conditions of Simulation. Wherever possible, filling trials should simulate the worst case. However, for initial validation of a new or modified filling machine or a new or modified facility, filling trials should be conducted independently from routine production, with filling lines set up specifically for the trial. For revalidation, trials should be done at the end of a normal filling operation when the risk of contamination due to accumulated errors is greatest and when operators are weariest. This is not possible for antibiotic products. In these cases the filling machine and the filling room must be cleaned free of antibiotic traces before conducting the filling trial to prevent bias in the results.

Before conducting a trial for initial validation purposes, all aspects of every aseptic control system should have been verified as meeting their validation standard. Microbiological monitoring above and beyond that normally expected should be done in the filling room before and after the filling trial.

The filling equipment should be set up according to its documented Standard Operating Procedure and run under normal operating conditions. Filling trials should be conducted by those personnel who are normally employed in the filling process. Ongoing revalidation filling trials should be seen as an opportunity to reinforce correct aseptic practices. Personnel should be dressed in normal aseptic filling room garments and perform routine production manipulations in response to events (sampling, check-weighing, etc.).

For liquid filling trials the containers need only be filled with sufficient media to wet all of the interior surfaces in a manner that simulates exposure in normal production. In other words, it is not necessary to simulate the exact volume of liquid filled in routine production. Indeed, exact simulation could create a quite impossibly large demand for sterile media beyond the capacity of labo ratory sterilizers. While suggesting this, it is important to recognize that every internal surface must come into contact with the medium. This may necessitate the incubation period being split into two halves, the first half with the containers incubated in their normal position, the second half with the containers incubated inverted.

Some companies do not sterilize media in the laboratory for filling trials. Instead they pass the media through the normal stages of sterile filtration applied to products being manufactured on the filling line. In this way they can economize on autoclave capacity while at the same time evaluating the aseptic manipulations associated with filtration. Although evaluation of these aseptic manipulations is essential to successful aseptic manufacture, the normal application of the filling trial is to the filling process alone. Aseptic manipulations associated with filtration and transfer are better evaluated independently, bringing greater focus on appropriate corrective action.

For solid dosage form filling trials, the final concentration of placebo in the microbiological growth medium should satisfy normal (pharmacopoeial) criteria for absence of growth inhibition. There are two approaches to the subsequent addition of microbiological media. The first is to have a liquid filler on line. This is the simplest and easiest of the two approaches, but it does run the risk of exposing solid dosage form filling personnel to an unfamiliar and potentially contaminating operation. Personnel must be specifically trained in running a trial in addition to their normal training required for solid dosage form filling. The second approach is to have the placebo-filled containers taken to a laboratory to be filled with media. This of course increases the risk of laboratory contamination and must be catered for by large-scale use of sterilized controls (often in a proportion of one control to two test containers).

Each filling trial should consist of at least 3000 items (it is normal practice to exceed the minimum to account for breakages, etc.). The medium of choice is *Soybean Casein Digest Broth USP.* Where necessary, for instance in antibiotic filling processes where, no matter how effective the cleaning, residues cannot be excluded, an inactivating agent (e.g., penicillinase) should be added to the medium at an appropriate concentration.

b. Interpretation of Results. After incubation, filled containers must be inspected and scored as sterile or nonsterile. Any contaminating microorganisms should be identified to at least generic level and where possible related to their most likely sources and to events occurring during the filling trial. The value of filling trial results is greatly enhanced by reliable knowledge of the time the items were being filled and the order in which they were filled.

The standard to be achieved is no more than one contaminated item in one thousand items. The FDA adds the proviso that this should be achieved to a 95% confidence level. What exactly does this mean? How should it be interpreted?

The PDA Technical Monograph on aseptic filling [19] quotes the following equation to describe the probability of finding one or more contaminated items in a sample of size N taken from a universe with a contamination rate of 0.1%:

$$P_{(x > 0)} = 1 - e^{-NP}$$

where $P_{(x > 0)}$ = the probability of detecting one or more contaminated items in the sample (for the purposes of the FDA's interpretation of filling trials this is equal to 95%), N = the number of items in the sample, and P = the probability of occurrence of contaminated items in the universe.

This equation describes an "operating characteristic" curve—the relationship between the percentage of contaminated items in the universe and the probability of accepting or rejecting the universe on the basis of finding at least one contaminated item in a sample of a specified size (N).

What this equation means in relation to filling trials is that if a series of samples each comprising 3000 items were taken from a universe that actually contained contaminated items at a frequency of one in one thousand (0.1%), we would find one or more contaminated items in 95% of our samples. It effectively defines a minimum sample size of 3000 (precisely 2996), because 95% confidence cannot be achieved with any smaller sample size. It also, by the inclusion of the expression $P_{(x > 0)}$, determines the pass/fail criterion as accept the universe with zero contaminated items in the sample, reject one or more contaminated items.

There are alternative interpretations of pass/fail criteria for filling trial results.

For instance, the proportion of contaminated items in a sample taken from a greater universe is not an exact measure of the proportion of contaminated items in the universe. It is only an estimate. For instance, one contaminated item in a sample of 3000 items provides an estimate (P_{est}) of 0.03% of the actual frequency of occurrence of contaminated items in the universe (P), which may be higher or lower than 0.03%. The reliability with which P_{est} can be claimed to reflect P can be calculated from the confidence limits of P_{est}.

Confidence limits may be calculated at 90% or 95% or whatever. For instance we can be 95% confident that P will lie between the lower and upper 95% confidence limits of P_{est}, etc.

If there is a large number of units in the sample (N) and P_{est} is not close to 0.5 (50%), confidence limits can be calculated according to the formula

$$P_{est} - \frac{hP_{est}Q_{est}}{N} < P < P_{est} + \frac{P_{est}Q_{est}}{N}$$

where h = the number of standard deviations appropriate to particular confidence limits (1.96 for 95%, 1.64 for 90% etc.), and

$$Q_{est} = 1 - P_{est}$$

In filling trials it is necessary (according to the FDA) to be 95% confident that P (the probability of contaminated units in the universe) is no greater than 0.001 (0.1%). Therefore 0.001 should be considered as the upper 95% confidence limit of P_{est}.

Table 6 lists the upper 95% confidence limits of P_{est} when P_{est} is one, two or three contaminated items in a sample of 3000 items (N). When P_{est} is 0.0003 (one contaminated item in three thousand), its upper 95% confidence limit is approximately 0.001 (0.1%). This interpretation therefore allows the pass/fail criterion for filling trials to be accept zero or one contaminated item, reject two or more contaminated items. The Table indicates the sample sizes that would be necessary to set the pass/fail criterion at two or less contaminated items (N = 5000) or three or less contaminated items (N = 7000). With three contaminated items in a sample of 3000 (P_{est} = 0.001) the upper confidence limit indicates that we cannot be 95% sure that P (the actual frequency of occurrence of contaminated items in the universe) is any less than 0.2%.

The third and least sophisticated approach to interpreting filling trial results is to regard the sample itself as the universe. This interpretation sets the pass/fail criterion at accept zero, one, two, or three contaminated items in three thousand, reject four or more.

In practice all three of these theoretical interpretations can be allied to the level of reaction required in response to filling trials.

No contaminated items in three thousand is the most favorable result that can be obtained from a filling trial. At initial validation of a new facility it should be interpreted as a cautious go-ahead signal as long as each and every

Table 6 Upper 95% Confidence Limits of P_{est} for Sample Sizes of 3000 to 7000

Number of contaminated items	Number of items in sample (N)				
	3000	4000	5000	6000	7000
1	0.10%	0.07%	0.06%	0.05%	0.04%
2	0.16%	0.12%	0.10%	0.08%	0.07%
3	0.21%	0.16%	0.13%	0.11%	0.09%

individual aseptic control system has been validated and confirmed to be satisfactory. At least two of the three replicate trials that are normally thought necessary for initial validations should have zero contaminated items; the third should be allowed to have no more than one contaminated item in the sample. Any other pattern of results should demand a thorough investigation, corrective action and, if necessary, revalidation before the facility is released for aseptic production.

With revalidation filling trials, zero contaminated items is once again a cautious go-ahead, and one contaminated item in 3000 should demand an investigation and appropriate corrective action where necessary while allowing production to continue. Two or three contaminated items should require any product manufactured on the filling line since the date of the failed trial to be quarantined until an investigation and a successful repeat trial has been completed.

More than three contaminated items in 3000 means a significant problem, in all likelihood compromising product sterility. The line or facility should be closed until all investigations, corrective actions, and satisfactory repeat trials have been completed. Product manufactured after the trial and before discovery of the failure should be considered for rejection unless there is a strong balance of evidence to support its release. If necessary, product manufactured before the trial should be considered for recall.

The translation of failed filling trial results to action against product is not an easy one for scientific, commercial, and pragmatic reasons. It may be six months since completion of the last successful filling trial and a great deal of product may be perceived to be at risk. The failure may be an isolated event due to an operator error; alternatively, it may signal a repeated problem that has previously gone unnoticed. Systematic equipment faults are easier to confirm and confine than systematic people faults.

Investigations should address the type of microorganisms isolated from the failed filling trial, their likely sources, their sensitivities to the antimicrobial characteristics of products that have been filled on the line, and most importantly their history of past occurrence. For instance, microorganisms that have been detected and represented as laboratory contamination in past Tests for Sterility should be considered as genuine product contaminants in those batches passed on retest. Batch withdrawal should be undertaken if they are also capable of surviving to any extent in the product. Identities should be at least to species level in failed filling trials.

7. Frequency of Revalidation: New aseptic manufacturing facilities and filling lines must be validated before they are allowed to be used for routine production. Thereafter, routine monitoring is a form of continuous abbreviated revalidation. However, the major validation activities are totally impossible when lines and facilities are operational. Revalidation and, if necessary, replacement of deteriorating equipment should be done at sufficiently frequent intervals to ensure continuing control. In practice the revalidation frequency is most often an operational compromise, typically twice per year during shutdowns.

B. Routine Monitoring of Aseptic Manufacturing Facilities

The purpose of routine monitoring of aseptic manufacturing facilities is to obtain some measure of the level of control being achieved. The ideal is that monitoring should be done in a way that will promptly reveal any failure of the control systems to meet their intended purpose. As often as not, practice falls somewhat short of this ideal.

The topics of how to monitor aseptic manufacturing environments, where to focus monitoring activities, how often to monitor, and what to do with the results are frequently debated. The regulatory literature is somewhat barren on those questions. For instance, the FDA's *Guideline on Sterile Drug Products Produced by Aseptic Processing* [2] deals with these topics in only slightly more than three pages of typescript; the "Orange Guide" [3] does so in four paragraphs. Industrial interest is reflected in two documents, one published by the Parenteral Society in the U.K. in 1989 [16], the other in the U.S. by the Parenteral Drug Association in 1990 [17]. Whereas these last two documents differ quite substantially in their treatment of environmental monitoring, their basic considerations remain as how, where, how often, and how to respond to environmental monitoring.

1. Methods for Environmental Monitoring: The methods available for monitoring aseptic manufacturing facilities are so well worn that even the regulatory documents are confident enough to recommend them. Microbiological air sampling (active and passive), microbiological surface sampling (swabs and contact plates), microbiological touch plates (finger dabs), physical particle monitoring, and monitoring of pressure differentials are the recommended approaches. Even so, there are many issues surrounding their use.

a. Measurement of Numbers of Microorganisms in Air. The "standard" active method uses a slit sampler. The principle of the slit sampler is that of inertial impaction; particles moving in an airstream have an individual inertia and may be deflected onto a surface where they may be trapped by impaction. Slit samplers (Fig. 17) are provided with pumps that draw air from the area being sampled through a narrow slit. The effect of the slit is to increase the velocity of the airflow and hence the inertial velocity of any particle being carried in the airstream. The accelerated particles are directed onto the surface of a plate of nutrient medium that is rotated continuously or progressively. Pumps provided with slit samplers usually operate at fixed rates, and the volume of air sampled is controlled by an on/off timer. Equipment suitable for use in connection with

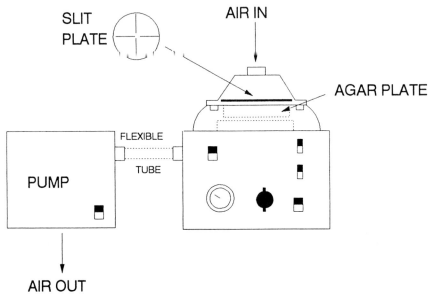

Fig. 17 Slit sampler.

aseptic filling rooms should consider pumping rates that allow 3.0 to 3.5 m^3 of air to be sampled in a reasonable time frame.

An alternative active air sampler is the centrifugal sampler (Fig. 18). Unlike the slit sampler, the centrifugal sampler is a neat lightweight sterilizeable instrument. This type of sampler uses centrifugation to remove particles from an airstream and trap them on agar strips. Centrifugal samplers have two technical problems. First, their sampling rates are low, too low to be sensitive enough to be of value in Class 100 clean rooms; second, the volume of air sampled is not accurately known [18], so they cannot legitimately be claimed to be quantitative devices.

The final method of air sampling is a passive one. This is the settle plate or fallout plate. Quite simply this is an agar plate left open and exposed for a specified period of time. Arguably this is as much a method of quantifying surface contamination as one of measuring air-borne contamination. As with many apparently simple methods, the settle plate represents a significantly complex equilibrium and results should be interpreted with great care.

Particles settle by gravity on to settle plates. Large and heavy particles tend to settle out due to gravitational forces; with increasing air movement only the very heaviest particles settle out. This limits the value of the method in laminar flow protected areas or other clean rooms where still air is not intended. Of course it can be argued that dead air is the main concern in clean rooms, and

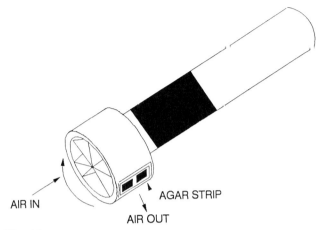

AIR IN

AGAR STRIP

AIR OUT

Fig. 18 Centrifugal air sampler.

settle plates are an effective method of detecting it. This argument depends on sitting the settle plate in the correct area, and it invites the question of why that location should be monitored with settle plates rather than corrected and then monitored by some better device.

The quantitative aspects of settle plates are debatable. What does one colony-forming unit represent? One viable microorganism? Or several microorganisms, perhaps up to a few hundred, carried on one large nonviable particle that has settled out? This rather restricts the quantitative value of settle plates, and some agencies concentrate only on their qualitative value, i.e., microorganisms identifiable as being of human origin, or microorganisms from air or dust or water, etc.

Some microorganisms may settle on settle plates and stay on the plates, while others may bounce off. What therefore is the settle plate an index of? Some microorganisms may remain viable on the plate but find the medium unsuitable for growth.

This is of course a problem common to all microbiological methodology. Other microorganisms may die on the surface of the plate. This introduces a long-standing debate concerning how long settle plates should be left exposed. Leaving them open too long leads to desiccation and death of the trapped microorganisms; if the plates are not exposed long enough the sensitivity of detection is diminished.

The Parenteral Drug Association [19] recommends 30 min for aseptic filling rooms; the Parenteral Society [16] recommends 4 h. Whyte and Niven [20] have argued that the viability on agar plates of microorganisms commonly found in room air is little affected by desiccation and quote allowable exposure periods of up to 24 h. There is no right answer to these problems. The time of exposure must be left to the discretion and professionalism of the microbiologist operating the monitoring program.

b. Measurement of Numbers of Microorganisms on Surfaces. There are two methods of monitoring surfaces, swabs and contact plates.

Swabbing is a technique in which a surface is lightly scrubbed with a moistened "collector" (swab), most often a cotton or alginate "bud." The swab is then rolled over the surface of an agar plate. Alternatively the swab may be immersed in a liquid and agitated to suspend the microorganisms collected. The liquid is then plated, or passed through a sterile membrane filter and plated on a nutrient medium.

The contact plate involves pressing an agar plate against the surface being monitored. The Rodac plate (diameter 55 mm) is a commercially available petri dish designed for use as a contact plate.

An important distinction is that the swab provides an index of the number of viable microorganisms contaminating an area of surface, whereas the contact plate provides an index of the number of contaminated sites within a particular area of surface.

The choice of which method to use, and where to use them, is debatable. Contact plates require that the surfaces that have been tested be thoroughly disinfected after testing to prevent traces of nutrient provoking microbiological growth where none might otherwise have occurred. Many workers believe that this is an unacceptable risk in connection with aseptic filling rooms but accept that the technique is useful in gray areas. Others reject contact plates completely, arguing that they are only suited to smooth plane surfaces, which by their nature are easily cleanable. Swabs have many advantages in this respect because they can be applied to surfaces that pose cleaning problems, for instance parts of machinery that are difficult to access but that may lead to significant product contamination.

c. Microbiological Touch Plates (Finger Dabs). Finger dabs are done by aseptic filling room personnel being required to press the tips of their fingers on to the surface of an agar plate. This is not really a method of monitoring the aseptic environment; it is either a method of monitoring the effectiveness of personnel discipline or a cosmetic exercise intended to reinforce aseptic practices.

d. Measurement of Numbers of Nonviable Particles in Air. The measurement of numbers of nonviable particles in air is an integral part of room classification at validation, and of course classification to clean room standards has a requirement for routine monitoring. The most widely used method is based on light scattering.

The principle is that an air sample is drawn into a sensor and passed through an area of intense light. Any particles in the airstream scatter the light. Thus the moving particles appear as bursts of light and can be detected with a photomultiplier or a photodiode. Each burst of light is converted into a pulse of electrical energy. The height of these pulses is proportional to the amount of light scattered by the particles. A digital counter sorts and counts the pulses according to their heights.

Two systems are available, polychromatic white light and lasers. Lasers are able to concentrate more energy in a smaller spot and are therefore able to register smaller particles. The lower limits of sensitivity for white light systems are in the order of 0.3 µm, and for lasers about 0.15 µm. For aseptic manufacturing facilities it is not normally necessary to measure particles smaller than 0.5 µm. Instruments should have the capability of sampling at least one ft^3 per minute.

Particle counters are not easily disinfected for taking into aseptic filling rooms. They may be dedicated to particular areas, or remote instruments with mobile or fixed sampling tubes can be purchased.

2. *Sample Location Selection*: Uniform contamination over a complete aseptic manufacturing facility is remotely improbable. It would require a total breakdown of systems and would be evident in many ways other than environmental monitoring. The selection of locations for environmental monitoring becomes therefore a matter of professional judgement that should take account of two major considerations: locations where, if contaminated, product quality would be most seriously affected; and locations that due to some vicissitude of design or control are susceptible to microbiological contamination or proliferation.

Monitoring of air for both viable and nonviable particles should be done in locations that reflect exposure of the dosage form to potential air-borne contamination. This usually means at or around table-top or machine-bed level with the sampling probes pointing vertically upward. It is not, however, necessary to monitor at the precise locations where dosage forms are actually exposed. In most instances it is better to choose indicator locations within filling rooms where the possibility of monitoring leading to product contamination is minimal. Air samplers themselves create air disturbance and movement that may disturb, deflect, or divert laminarity, cause momentary localized dead space, or unbalance pressure differentials. There is a major dilemma to be resolved in every choice of air sampling location: the choices are between the combination of the most relevant monitoring location with potential compromise of control, and the combination of an indicator location with less relevance to product contamination coupled with no compromise of control. Most pragmatists choose the latter.

If surface-to-surface contamination is potentially more significant than air-borne contamination, as many aseptic filling operators now believe, then touch plates (finger dabs) become a critical part of environmental monitoring. Not so much does their value lie in whether they indicate contamination or absence of contamination but in the identification of contaminants to their most likely source. Touch plates should be seen as a route to identifying systems failure and can be truly relevant to product contamination. Within aseptic filling rooms, personnel should be required to disinfect their hands thoroughly after touch plate impressions have been taken to ensure that traces of media remaining do not lead to microbial proliferation in the filling room.

Surface samples should not be so concentrated on direct relevance that they lead to unnecessary intrusions into critical filling zones. It is best that within white areas they concentrate on locations that are difficult to access for cleaning and locations where manual operations are routinely carried out. The purpose of these choices is again to expose systems failures.

Surface monitoring can be very important in gray areas. Identification of failure of control systems implies investigation and correction. Once a white area has been cleaned and fumigated, with modern HEPA filtration systems the most likely route of entry of contaminants is via the gray areas. Discipline is not expected to be as severe in these areas. There may be water, sinks, clean rather than sterile equipment, clean rather than sterile clothing, etc. In changing rooms there may be opportunity for cross contamination of dedicated clothing with street clothes. The possibilities for introducing routes of contamination are legion. The choice of locations for routine environmental monitoring in these areas should concentrate very heavily on locations that may lead to microbial proliferation.

The choice of locations should be documented but should not be too rigid. There are several reasons for this. First, environmental monitoring assistants should not feel so confined to a mechanical task that they fail to notice vulnerabilities or lapses in control. The trained and discriminating human eye is a better environmental monitoring method than any of the formal systems described above. Second, filling personnel should not become conditioned to cleaning and disinfecting monitoring locations at the expense of other locations. It is all to easy in routine environmental monitoring to condition employees to bad habits rather than good ones.

3. Frequency of Environmental Sampling: Environments become sterile through being cleaned, decontaminated, and sterilized. The maintenance of sterility is achieved through a series of control systems that overlap and back up one another. These systems for maintaining asepsis operate continuously. Their effectiveness at maintaining asepsis is monitored on the same basis as any other continuous process. The aseptic environment cannot be batched into neat day-sized or week-sized chunks that can be sampled, tested, and classified as accept/reject on the basis of the results. The frequency of environmental monitoring should not therefore be set as a simple function of time, daily, weekly, etc.

In the absence of reliable data indicating a history of control for an aseptic manufacturing facility, it is good sense to list all those events that might have a deleterious effect on the provision of an aseptic environment (batch changes, shift changes, process interruptions, etc.). The environment should at first be monitored at a frequency that will confirm or contradict the hypothesis that change has a significant deleterious effect on the aseptic environment.

Particular attention should be given to any buildup of contamination that may arise between major clean-downs/decontaminations. If buildup should arise it may be necessary to improve the cleaning methods, improve the environmental controls, or shorten the interval between clean-downs/decontaminations.

When there is enough reliable data to discriminate between significant changes and insignificant changes arising from scheduled, routine, predictable events, and to support the interval of time between clean-downs/decontaminations, the environmental monitoring program can be addressed as a function of time.

The assumption that is being made when it comes to interpreting results is that the quality of the environment between two successive monitorings does not differ from the quality measured at each time of monitoring.

4. Responding to Monitoring Data: Data from routine environmental monitoring programs are not sufficient on their own to certify that all processes and conditions that might influence the sterility of products manufactured in the aseptic facility are satisfactory and under control. They are only one part of the overall system of sterility assurance.

Data should be evaluated to discern any change (improvement or deterioration) to the level of control existing in an area or at a location. Limits should be set and any excursions beyond those limits should demand a formal response. Each location should be addressed separately for these purposes. Progressive change within these limits should also be reviewed in an attempt to predict improvement or deterioration.

Limits should be set carefully. Table 7 identifies some limits that have been proposed. Microbiological test methods are generally less sensitive than chemical or physical methods and are vulnerable to limits being exceeded by accidental contamination that does not necessarily relate to the aseptic manufacturing environment. Almost every textbook, laboratory manual, and methods guide to microbiology contains a statement that plates for colony counting should contain when possible 30 to 300 colonies. Environmental monitoring limits for aseptic environments are typically well short of these numbers.

For most microbiological purposes plates with counts within proposed environmental limits would be rejected on the basis of chance contamination (were it to have arisen) having an unacceptably high proportional effect on the result.

Microbiological methods are separately too insensitive to detect fluctuations in environmental control that could be significant to the sterility of aseptically filled products. In combination they are a more powerful tool, because the probability of two or three independent methods being subject to simultaneous chance contamination becomes rapidly more remote.

Table 7 Proposed [16,17] Target Levels for Environmental Monitoring of Aseptic Manufacturing Facilities

Test method	White area	Grey areas
Settle plates	< 5 cfu per 90 mm plate; exposure 4 h	< 40 cfu per 90 mm plate; exposure 4 h
Active air samples	< 10 cfu per m³ (equivalent to < 3 per 10 ft³) < 1 cfu per 10 ft³ (equivalent to < 3.5 per m³)	< 80 cfu per m³ (equivalent to < 25 per 10 ft³)
Surface samples	< 5 cfu per 0.0024 m³ (equivalent to a Rodac Plate)	< 80 cfu per 0.0024 m³ (equivalent to a Rodac Plate)
Touch plates	< 1 cfu per 5 fingers	< 5 cfu per 5 fingers

V. CONTAMINATION CONTROL FOR TERMINALLY STERILIZED PRODUCTS

Some or all of the principles of aseptic manufacture are used in the manufacture of terminally sterilized products. There are two main reasons for this. The first is microbiological. The numbers and types of microorganisms present in or on a product item prior to sterilization make up a major determinant of sterility and merit serious consideration. The second reason is the avoidance of large nonviable particles in parenteral products.

There is substantial evidence (much from the literature on drug abuse) indicating that particulate matter (undissolved substances) is a health hazard in parenteral products [21]. The precise hazards depend very much on the physical and biological properties of the particles, and their site of lodgement in the vascular system. Phlebitis and pulmonary infarctions are the most significant problems associated with particulate matter. Particulate matter is an unwanted and unnecessary addition to parenteral therapy.

Terminally sterilized parenteral products are therefore usually manufactured under conditions very similar or even identical to those of aseptic manufacture.

The sources of particulate matter are packaging components, manufacturing conditions, and formulation components. The mechanisms of controlling particles in all of these categories have already been alluded to earlier in this chapter. Their control is through the same mechanisms described for the control of microbiological contamination. The washing processes for glass product contact containers and rubber closures are more related to removal of spicules and elastomeric fragments than to the removal of microbiological contamination. Pressurized air and laminar flow control both microbial and particulate contamination from the manufacturing process. The choice of materials for manufacturing equipment should consider their potential to contribute particles to the product. Filters capable of removing microbiological particles are also capable of removing potentially hazardous larger nonviable particles.

Pharmacopoeial limits for nonviable particles in large-volume parenteral products have been long established. The USP introduced standards for small-volume parenterals in 1985.

This standard for small-volume parenterals was set at 20% of that for large volume parenterals on the unfounded assumption that the average patient receives five small-volume parenterals for each single large-volume infusion.

There are no compendial standards to limit particulate matter in the devices used for delivery of parenteral products to the patient. In-line filters are being increasingly included in infusion sets and devices.

Microbiological control and particulate control go hand in hand in the technology of aseptic manufacture. Microbiological control of medical devices prior to terminal sterilization rarely requires such intense effort or as much capital investment.

Many medical products and their processes of manufacture are innately particle generating. For instance, with cellulosic materials used for manufacture of sterile dressings it is impossible to avoid both particulate and microbiological contamination. With plastic medical devices the situation is different. The conditions of pressure and temperature at which plastics are molded or extruded are sufficient to sterilize such components at the point of manufacture. On the other hand, these processes are significantly particle generating. There is little point in endeavoring to operate most medical device manufacturing processes in the same type of clean room conditions used for aseptic manufacture; they would be impossible to achieve.

The concentration of effort in contamination control for sterile medical devices is therefore toward controlling the major sources of both microbiological and particulate contamination but without specific targets. There is no regulatory necessity to manufacture medical devices in classified clean rooms, although Class 100,000 may be achievable in many processes. The requirement is for a controlled manufacturing area with intact floors, walls, and ceilings, for controlled access (personnel and raw materials) and egress (personnel, finished product, and waste), and for high standards of personal hygiene.

The process of injection molding, for instance, produces a sterile product at point of manufacture as stated above. Molding polymers are, however, particulate in nature. The raw material may lead to higher than necessary particulate contamination.

This is best controlled by operating a centralized polymer room separated from the molding process and capable of delivering the polymer to the molding machine through a sealed system. The amount of vibration arising from the operation of molding machines is innately particle generating. The mechanism of removing molded components from their sprue or runner may also be particle generating (this is best done automatically but in some instances may require manual intervention).

Collection of molded components should be in sterile nonparticle shedding plastics. Robotic devices can be used to remove easily deformable components from the mold face and transfer them gently to receptacles. Wooden pallets should be avoided. There is no fundamental reason why injection molding processes should not operate in the total absence of personnel. The ideal is not often achieved.

Thereafter, contamination of medical devices assembled from molded plastic components is very much a function of their exposure to personnel. Superb air quality is not required, so some base level of contamination as a result of its absence is inevitable. Personnel should be trained in hygiene and equipped with nonshedding overalls (usually smocks with high collars and fitted wrists), headcovers, and shoe covers. Gloves are not usually a consideration for medical device manufacture unless for some particularly critical operation or a very tightly specified sterilization process. In general terms, the level of microbiological contamination found on medical devices prior to sterilization has a crude inverse relationship to the extent of automation used in the device's assembly. It is paradoxical however that the amount of particulate contamination tends to increase with automation due to the vibration from machinery.

The manufacture of terminally sterilized medical and pharmaceutical products is controlled therefore to minimize microbiological and particulate contamination. There is a major divide separating the conditions necessary for parenteral products from conditions satisfactory for nonparenteral products. Irrespective of whether they are being aseptically manufactured or terminally sterilized, the manufacture of parenteral products requires superbly controlled and monitored manufacturing conditions. This is in the main because of the need to control nonviable particulate contamination as well as microbiological contamination. For medical devices, where particulate contamination is unavoidable, the need is only to control microbiological contamination. The requirement at best is about the same as the requirement for controlling gray aseptic manufacturing areas, but for the most part it is a good deal less stringent.

REFERENCES

1. Whyte, W., and Donaldson, N. (1989). Cleaning a cleanroom. *Medical Device and Diagnostic Industry* **11** (2): 31–35.
2. Food and Drug Administration (1987). *Guideline on Sterile Drug Products Produced by Aseptic Processing.* Washington, D.C.
3. Her Majesty's Stationery Office (1983). *Guide to Good Manufacturing Practice.* London.
4. Commission of the European Communities (1992). *The Rules Governing Medicinal Products in the European Community, Volume 4, Guide to Good Manufacturing*

Practice for Medicinal Products. Luxembourg: Office for Official Publications of the European Communities.

5. Federal Standard 209B (1976). *Clean Room and Work Station Requirements. Controlled Environment.* Washington, D.C.: General Services Administration.
6. Federal Standard 209D (1988). *Clean Room and Work Station Requirements. Controlled Environment.* Washington, D.C.: General Services Administration.
7. British Standards Institution (1976). *Environmental Cleanliness in Enclosed Spaces. Part 1. Specification for Controlled Environment Clean Rooms, Work Stations and Clean Air Devices.* BS 5295: Part 1. London: Her Majesty's Stationery Office.
8. British Standards Institution (1989). *Environmental Cleanliness in Enclosed Spaces. Part 0. General Introduction, Terms and Definitions for Clean Rooms and Clean Air Devices.* BS 5295: Part 0. *Part 1. Specifications for Clean Rooms and Clean Air Devices.* BS 5295: Part 1. *Part 2. Specifications for Monitoring Clean Rooms and Clean Air Devices to Prove Continued Compliance with BS 5295: Part 1.* BS 5295: Part 2. London: Her Majesty's Stationery Office.
9. Sharp, J. R. (1987). Manufacture of sterile pharmaceutical products using "blow-fill-seal" technology. *Pharmaceutical Journal* **239**: 106–108.
10. Sharp, J. R. (1988). Validation of a new form-fill-seal installation. *Manufacturing Chemist*, February 1988, 22–23, 27, 55.
11. Bradley, A., Probert, S. P., Sinclair, C. S., and Tallentire, A. (1991). Airborne microbial challenges of blow/fill/seal equipment: A case study. *Journal of Parenteral Science and Technology* **45**: 187–192.
12. Fry, E. M. (1983). Aseptic processing of pharmaceutical products—Regulatory considerations. In *Proceedings of National Food Processors Association Conference,* October 11-12, 1983, Washington, D.C.
13. Whyte, W. (1981). Settling and impaction of particles into containers in manufacturing pharmacies. *Journal of Parenteral Science and Technology* **35**: 255.
14. National Conference of Standards Laboratories (1986). *Recommended Practice. Medical Products and Pharmaceutical Industry Calibration Control System.*
15. American Society for Testing Materials (1973). ASTM F 51/68.
16. Parenteral Society (1990). *Technical Monograph No. 2. Environmental Contamination Control Practice.* Swindon, U.K.: Parenteral Society.
17. PDA Environmental Task Force (1990). Technical Report No. 13 Fundamentals of a microbiological environmental monitoring program. *Journal of Parenteral Science and Technology* **44**: S1–S16.
18. Kaye, S. (1988). Efficiency of "Biotest RCS" as a sampler of airborne bacteria. *Journal of Parenteral Science and Technology* **42**: 147–152.
19. PDA (1980). *Technical Monograph No. 2. Validation of Aseptic Filling for Solution Drug Products.* Philadelphia: Parenteral Drug Association.
20. Whyte, W., and Niven, L. (1987) Airborne bacteria sampling: The effect of dehydration and sampling time. *Journal of Parenteral Science and Technology* **40**: 182–188.
21. Borchert, S. J., Abe, A., Aldrich, D. S., Fox, L. E., Freeman, J. E., and White, R. D. Particulate matter in parenteral products: A review. *Journal of Parenteral Science and Technology* **40**: 212–241.
22. Federal Standard 209E (1992). *Airborne Particulate Cleanliness Classes in Cleanrooms and Clean Zones.* Washington, D.C.: General Services Administration.

9
Maintenance of Sterility

The sterile condition can only exist within barriers that protect it from the non-sterile general environment. An essential prerequisite to the maintenance of sterility is for the product or part of the product that is required to be sterile to be isolated by containment within a material impermeable to microbial penetration. If the design of the containment system or primary package does not allow the material of containment to be continuous, all-enveloping, and complete, then the sealing surfaces of the material of containment, either to itself or to another material of containment or to the product itself, must also be impermeable to microbial penetration. The barrier properties of the containment system to microbial penetration must be sufficient to withstand the rigors of sterilization and tolerant to extreme conditions of transportation and storage throughout the product's shelf-life. Yet containment should not be so secure that it becomes impossible to use the product without compromising its sterility.

Some systems of containment for sterile medical and pharmaceutical products have become so widely used that expectation has become conditioned to their being the systems of first choice. Sterile pharmaceuticals are expected to be contained in glass, mainly in the form of bottles, ampoules, or vials, but also in other presentations such as prefilled syringes. Glass has achieved its predominance through an extensive body of knowledge confirming its inertness and compatibility with pharmaceutically active substances. It is also impermeable to microorganisms and stable at thermal sterilization temperatures. Other materials such as plastics are also used for sterile pharmaceuticals, but not so extensively. Medical devices are expected to be contained within flexible packaging, most often nowadays consisting of polymeric film material, but originating from the tolerance of particular types of microbiologically impermeable paper to steam, gas, and radiation sterilization.

I. CONSIDERATIONS FOR CONTAINMENT OF STERILE PRODUCTS

The choice of appropriate containment systems for maintaining sterility is particular to specific products. It may often be rather complex. Factors relating to the materials of containment and to the overall system of containment should be considered separately and then in combination to achieve the best end result.

A. Materials of Containment

Some of the major factors affecting the choice of materials of containment include

(a) Microbiological impermeability. Materials that are impermeable to molecular migration such as glass are guaranteed to be impermeable to microbiological penetration. Some forms of flexible packaging are deliberately chosen to allow the passage of steam or ethylene oxide gas. These materials must be evaluated specifically for their impermeability to microbial penetration. In this respect their properties can be compared directly to the properties of filter media.

(b) Biological properties of the material. Materials should not leach biologically active substances into or onto the product. In some instances this may be a simple decision; in others it may require knowledge of the behavior of the material in relation to the specific product. In general terms, pharmaceutical types of glass do not pose problems of a biological nature.

(c) Chemical properties of the material. Materials should not leach chemical impurities into or onto the product. These properties should not be worsened by sterilization treatment nor by storage over time.

(d) Suitability of the material for sterilization. Sterile products cannot be allowed to come into contact with nonsterile containment materials. The materials of containment must therefore be able to retain all of their favorable properties in the face of the rigors of a sterilization process. Most types of glass turn brown when irradiated; clear glass and irradiation sterilization are therefore incompatible. Impermeable materials are incompatible with ethylene oxide sterilization. Heat-labile materials are incompatible with thermal sterilization.

(e) Strength of the material. Will the material withstand transportation and storage? Glass is fragile. Paper tears easily. It may well be that some other properties outweigh strength considerations, or that lack of strength of the material may be compensated for in the overall design of the containment system, or that there may be protection afforded to a fragile material by secondary packaging required for other purposes like ease of handling during shipment. Innovation may lead to development of materials that improve upon the strength of traditional materials while retaining their benefits, for instance in the way that spun-bonded polyolefins improve upon paper.

(f) Printability of the material. Can the material be printed to identify its contents, or to provide instructions on its use? This may often be a most important consideration. An unidentified pharmaceutical or medical product is a serious hazard to the unsuspecting user. Printing should not be thought to be restricted to opaque materials; glass ampoules may carry instructions in ceramic print or may be ring coded to identify their contents.

B. Systems of Containment

The overall system of containment may consist of more than one material of containment. Glass ampoules are the most obvious example of a single-material containment system. Vials consist of a glass container and a rubber or polymeric closure. Some device packages may have one side consisting of an opaque material printed with instructions for use and the other side of a transparent material allowing the consumer to see the contents. For systems of containment an extra dimension of complexity is introduced into the most important of the factors affecting materials, their microbiological impermeability. The extra dimension is the microbiological integrity of the overall system and particularly in relation to sealing one material surface to another.

The choice of a system of containment must address the following major factors relating to container-closure integrity:

(a) Microbiological impermeability of the seal. How are surfaces sealed one to another? Molecular bonding is the method of choice, for instance in heat-sealed glass ampoules, and in heat-sealing paper to paper, paper to polymeric film, or polymeric film to polymeric film. Dimensional inter-ference fit, for instance between the outside neck diameter of a closure and the inside neck diameter of a vial, is an acceptable alternative. Adhesives may also produce microbiologically impermeable seals.

(b) Suitability for sterilization. Will the seal break down when sterilized? Will internal headspace pressure in autoclaving vials blow the closures out? Will the pressure differentials in ethylene oxide sterilization burst flexible packaging seals open?

(c) Seal strength. This is a curiously ambiguous property. Seals should be strong enough to maintain microbiological integrity through sterilization (if considering a terminal process), transportation, and storage. On the other hand they usually constitute the route whereby the product is removed for use, so they should not be too difficult to open.

Other aspects of the overall systems of containment for sterile products include the shape and size of the system. These factors may affect its fragility, the ways in which the product may be sterilized, and the ways in which the product itself may be removed from its containment system. The potential for movement of the product within its containment system should be restricted if damage and potential loss of sterility are to be avoided.

Clearly, containment systems must be specified in some detail with regard to those properties that may affect their resistance to microbiological penetration. For simple systems such as rubber stoppered glass vials, dimensional specifica-tions should address the internal diameter of the neck opening and its depth, the internal and external diameters of the flange, and the concentricity of the flange, the neck, and the body of the vial. Any angularity of the flange versus the verti-cal center line of the vial must be specified; so must the physical finish of the surfaces of flange and internal neck bore to ensure satisfactory mating with the closure. Closures should be specified in terms of diameters, depth, thickness, and elasticity.

Other containment systems must be specified in similar levels of detail if there is to be consistent assurance of maintenance of microbiological integrity.

II. MICROBIOLOGICAL EVALUATION OF MAINTENANCE OF STERILITY

A microbiologically contaminated product is nonsterile regardless of the manner in which the contamination arose. Nonsterility may have arisen through an inadequate sterilization process, through contamination during aseptic processing, or through failure of the system of containment. Systems of containment should therefore, like all other systems contributing to the assurance of sterility, be shown to be capable of meeting their intended purpose, i.e., to maintain sterility.

It may be obvious that a containment system has failed to maintain sterility. The contents of a broken ampoule have no assurance of sterility. A syringe received in an open package cannot be supposed to be sterile. Other deficiencies in containment systems may pose greater threats to the user of the medical or pharmaceutical product because they go unnoticed. It is these more subtle problems that demand serious consideration.

Microbiological evaluation ought to be done as part of the validation program for new or changed containment systems or new or changed materials of containment. Physical or chemical testing is best used for routine purposes if it can be assumed that these characteristics relate to the microbiological barrier properties of the containment system. There are two broad systems in use for microbiologically evaluating barrier properties of materials. These are microbiological immersion challenge methods and microbiological aerosol challenge methods [1]. The microorganisms differ within each type of test, and between tests; there is no accepted standard method, and details differ from one laboratory to another.

A. Microbiological Immersion Challenge Tests

The microbiological immersion challenge test is probably the most severe test of containment system integrity. The test accepts that microbiological penetration into a container is most likely to occur in the event of a continuous film or bridge of liquid forming between the general contaminated environment and the contained protected environment. To a large extent it mimics the possibility of the containment system becoming wetted in transport, storage, or use. Wetting may arise from sources within the containment system, e.g., a liquid formulation leaking out of a vial, or from outside the containment system, e.g., splashing, rainwater, condensation. Immersion is probably the most appropriate test method for rigid containment systems, for containment systems containing liquids, and for any type of product where wetting might arise but not be immediately or obviously apparent.

Frieben et al. [2] filled vials with *Soybean Casein Digest Medium,* sealed them, and then immersed them inverted in a suspension of 10^8 *Escherichia coli* per mL for 10 min. Other sources are quoted [3] to use *Serratia marcescens* at 10^6 per mL for 30 min contact time.

The factors that might lead to microorganisms breaching the microbiological integrity of practical containment systems are not well defined. Some workers using *Pseudomonas diminuta* believe that motility and size may be of critical importance; the nature of the liquid carrier and its contact angle with the containment system may also contribute. The Parenteral Drug Association [1] acknowledges that this test may be made more sensitive by increasing the level of stress on the system by using dynamic changes in temperature and pressure. Satisfactory microbiological challenge test data from respectable sample sizes and against severe challenges provide good assurance of maintenance of sterility.

A rigorous approach to microbiological immersion challenge testing is depicted in Fig. 1. This method uses *Pseudomonas diminuta* grown in Lactose Broth at 31°C for 24 h. The culture is then sonicated before use to break up any microcolonies or rosettes that may have arisen and that may reduce the potential for this microorganism to penetrate across tiny flaws in intended microbial barriers.

The test procedure is carried out over 5 days, and incubation continues for 14 more. In the first stage of the test, media-filled containers are immersed inverted into the culture of *Ps. diminuta* for 10 s to a depth where the container/closure interface is completely covered. The containers are then incubated at 31°C for 24 h. Next day the procedure is repeated, but incubation of the containers over the second 24 h period is at 5°C. The third and fourth days of the trial follow the same procedure of immersion and incubation, but the containers are inverted during incubation. After immersion on the fifth day, the containers are incubated in their normal configuration at 31°C for a further 14 days.

This type of procedure is intended to exaggerate the conditions that might lead to microbiological penetration of containment systems. For instance, inverted incubation is intended to encourage liquid contact with the container/closure interface, whereas there may normally be some headspace separating the two in the containers' normal configuration. Incubation at alternating temperatures of 31°C and 5°C is intended to exaggerate any tendency toward expansion and contraction of the materials of the microbiological containment system that may encourage the formation of liquid bridges between the exterior and the interior.

Microbiological approaches such as that described above are very evidently laborious, time-consuming, and unsuited to routine use. Dye penetration may be substituted for microbiological immersion challenge testing in routine use.

B. Microbiological Aerosol Challenge Tests

If it can be safely assumed that the packaged product is not going to come into contact with water, either as outward leakage or from inward contamination, it is

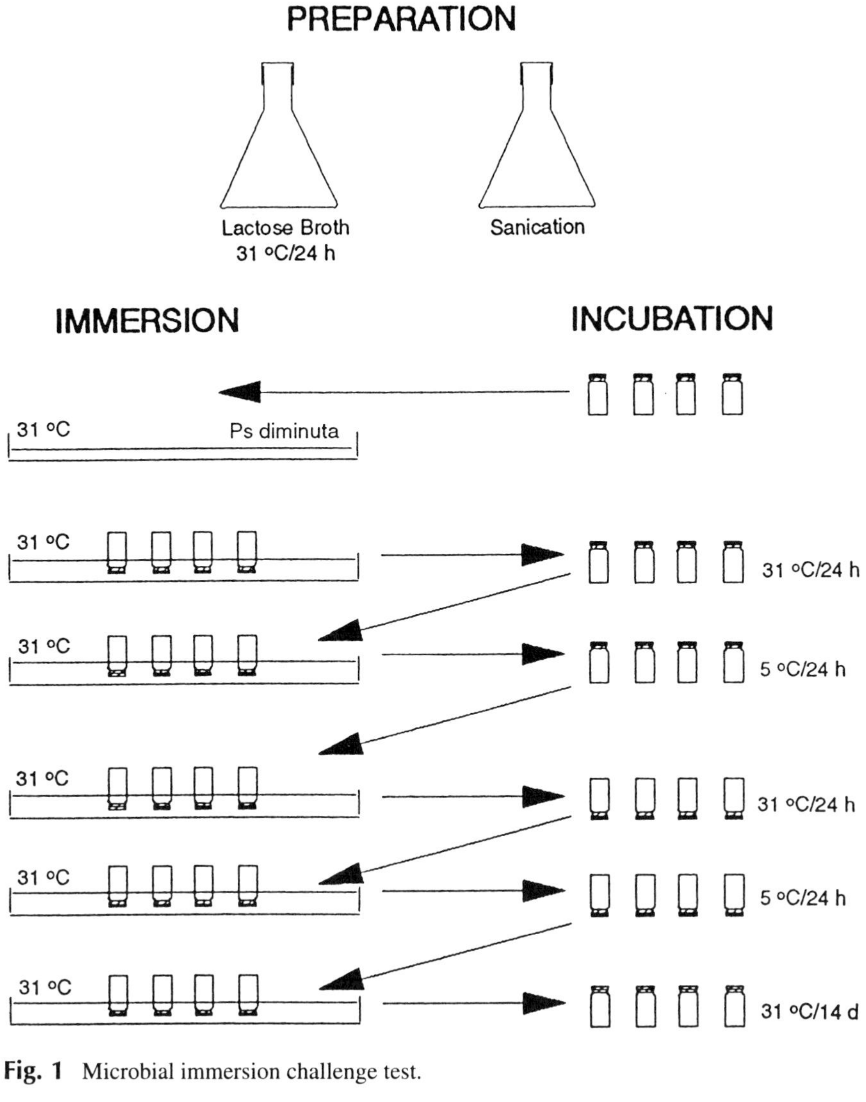

PREPARATION

Lactose Broth
31 °C/24 h

Sanication

IMMERSION   INCUBATION

Fig. 1 Microbial immersion challenge test.

probably inappropriately severe to test the containment system by an immersion test.   In these cases microbiological aerosol challenges mimic reality more closely.   The scope of aerosol testing is only limited by the technology chosen. The choice and concentration of microorganisms in the challenge is also only a function of the technology and the chosen severity of the challenge.

Microbiological aerosol challenges are particularly appropriate for the types of flexible packaging used for medical devices. There is rarely any liquid content to leak out. External water damage is often obvious and should stimulate rejection of the product. On the other hand, there is a real risk of unnoticeable air-borne microorganisms passing through pinholes in the material or through the seals of flexible containment systems. The risk of failure to provide satisfactory containment may be increased if temperature or pressure differentials between the air within the package and the general environment give rise to forces that may drive microorganisms inward. Some flexible packaging materials, for instance those used in connection with radiation sterilization, can be totally impermeable to molecular movement; others, for instance those used in connection with ethylene oxide and steam sterilization, must be permeable (or have permeable inserts) to molecular movement. The risk of encountering pinholes is greatest in these permeable materials.

Powell [4] recommended the use of an aerosol suspension of *Serratia marcescens* in a respirator to test product-filled sealed flexible packages. The packages were subjected to alternative positive and negative pressures at a frequency of 20 cycles per min over 2 h duration to simulate the changes in environmental temperature and pressure that might be encountered in transport and storage. On completion of the challenge the contents of the package were tested for sterility. This is a relatively unsophisticated system.

Experimental technologies become more elaborate as they attempt to address some of the uncontrolled variables present in the type of test described by Powell [4], typically

(a) Maintenance of viability. Some microorganisms may have only limited viability in aerosol suspension and thus could provide a falsely high impression of the severity of the challenge. Better experimental technologies allow periodic withdrawal of samples from the aerosol to check viability.

(b) Humidity. The two major reasons for wishing to control humidity are first because of the effects of humidity on microbiological viability (most microorganisms naturally encountered in atmospheric air are resistant to desiccation but many others are highly sensitive to dry conditions) and second to simulate the effects of moist atmospheric conditions on the barrier properties of the containment system.

(c) Homogeneity of the suspension. It is sensible to prevent the microorganisms from settling out of suspension during the challenge period. This is normally done by maintaining air movement by fans or by recirculation during the challenge.

(d) Uniformity of particle size. Uniform particle sizes are most usually obtained by nebulizing the microbial suspension into the challenge chamber.

(e) Qualitative or quantitative penetration. The amount of information obtainable from quantal response experiments (penetration or no penetration) is limited. For experimental purposes that attempt to relate physical characteristics of the containment material or containment system it is necessary to obtain quantitative data. This may be done by arranging to collect and cultivate those microorganisms that penetrate the barrier systems.

One such system recommended for packaging films by Reich [5] described a challenge of *Bacillus subtilis* atomized via a Devilbiss nebulizer into a test chamber to a concentration of 10^4 spores per m^3. The spores were maintained in homogeneous suspension by means of a fan, and the chamber was equipped with a pump to allow pressure differentials to be created across the samples of material under test. The test films are situated over bacteria-retentive membranes to allow quantitative comparison of various pressure differentials and flow rates. Other elaborate experimental technologies include those of Tallentire and Sinclair [6]; using spores of *Bacillus subtilis* var *niger* these workers showed significant differences in microbiological penetration through paper and spun-bonded polyolefin webs over flow rates from 1 to 100 cm^3 per min per cm^2.

The same principles of controlled aerosol challenge can be applied to sealed packages, except that flow into sealed packs is far more difficult to achieve than flow across samples of films or webs. It is very doubtful, also, whether this type of aerosol testing can be meaningfully applied to rigid containment systems. It is unlikely that aerosols can pose a severe challenge to say glass vials with oversealed rubber closures. Toward the end of the nineteenth century Pasteur demonstrated the intrinsic unlikelihood of air-borne microorganisms traversing a convoluted pathway in the absence of some specific driving force to contaminate nutrient infusions. It is similarly unlikely for microorganisms to traverse a tortuous channel between an elastomeric closure and a glass flange.

III. PHYSICAL EVALUATION OF MAINTENANCE OF STERILITY

Physical evaluation of the containment systems used in the maintenance of sterility is an acceptable alternative to microbiological evaluation, because it is the integrity of physical systems that creates barriers to microbiological penetration of containment materials and systems. For instance, a pinhole in a flexible package or a crack in a glass vial is a loss of integrity of the containment system; the fact that microorganisms can theoretically traverse that crack or pinhole is sufficient to compromise sterility without having to set out specifically to demonstrate that this is so by microbiological methodology. Physical test methods are almost always simpler and less expensive than microbiological methods. Some may correlate with microbiological characteristics, some may be nondestructive, some may even be suited to 100% inspection.

The types of physical evaluation that are available are quite product specific, and technical details vary extensively. Some examples relating to commonly used systems of containment are described below.

A. Glass Ampoules

There is no need to demonstrate repeatedly that microorganisms are unable to penetrate the molecular structure of glass. Ideally, ampoules present a hermetic environment totally enclosed within glass. A completely broken ampoule is obvious, and more than likely its contents have spilled or leaked out. The subtlety of inadequate ampoules is in tiny cracks through which microorganisms may penetrate and, more likely, unsatisfactory flame sealing of the ampoule.

The traditional approach to evaluating the integrity of ampoules has been through 100% inspection by a vacuum dye penetration test. The basic procedure for the vacuum dye penetration test is to place racks of sealed ampoules in a dye bath, apply a vacuum for a period of time, remove and rinse the ampoules, and then inspect for dye penetration.

Dye solutions should be chosen with some care; they should be easily washable from the ampoule surfaces after the test and should not be toxic in the event of unsatisfactory washing; they should also have a high color intensity or fluorescence, and these properties should not be lost by interaction with the ampoule contents.

Typical dye bath tests begin by placing the ampoules under test in a chamber, evacuating the chamber to about 0.85 bar, and holding for 10 to 15 min. The dye is then admitted to the chamber and the chamber pressure increased to about 2 bar and held for a further 10 to 15 min. The ampoules are then washed, dried, and inspected. Inspection is most often visual but may be done by automated optical detection methods.

Dye immersion is not, however, theoretically sound with respect to detecting microbial penetration.

The amount of fluid that can enter a circular pore is governed by Poiseuille's law:

$$t = \frac{8 \cdot l \cdot V \cdot n}{\pi \cdot r^4 \cdot dP}$$

where t = the minimum time required for volume V to penetrate a capillary, V = the volume penetrating in time t, n = the viscosity of the fluid, l = length of the capillary, r = radius of the capillary, and dP = pressure differential across the capillary.

If it is to be considered that microorganisms can penetrate capillaries with diameters as small as 0.4 μm (and this is a reasonable assumption, because *Pseudomonas diminuta* was first encountered from having passed through filter membranes with 0.45 μm pore size ratings), Poiseuille's law can be used to calculate the dimensions of a satisfactory vacuum dye penetration test.

Given ampoules with wall thicknesses of 4×10^{-2} cm, methylene blue with a viscosity of 10^{-2} poise in 1% solution, and a pressure differential of 2×10^6 dyn/cm, the minimum time required for 10^{-5} mL (a reasonable guess at the minimum perceptible volume) to penetrate through a 0.4 μm pinhole would be 9 h. Practical testing times in the vacuum dye penetration test are in the region of 15 min.

A further complication in relation to the dye penetration test is the possibility of microbiologically contaminated dye penetrating some of the ampoules and going unnoticed during inspection. Sterile dye solutions are usually specified for this test.

An alternative to the dye test is high-voltage electronic pinhole detection. The subjectivity of visual inspection is eliminated, the time taken to complete the test is shorter, and it is usually automated and can be run as a continuous inspection system rather than as a batchwise inspection system. Ampoules are individually exposed to a high-frequency voltage. Ohm's law dictates that the current flowing in the system is proportional to the voltage applied and inversely proportional to the resistance of the system. Glass has insulating properties that when intact confer high resistance to the flow of current. Pinholes or cracks in the glass, and even regions of thinner than normal glass, allow the discharge current to enter the ampoule; the resistance of the system decreases measurably, and the resultant signal can be channelled into automatic rejection of the corresponding ampoule. Sensitivity to 0.5 μm is claimed.

High-voltage methods are not restricted to glass ampoules; indeed, they may be used for other materials with high resistances such as plastics, and for other types of containers such as vials.

B. Glass Vials with Elastomeric Closures

There is a United States Federal Specification dated 1976 that describes a physical test for vial integrity consisting of suspending the vials upside down at room temperature for 2 h and then at 49°C for 4 h. Evidence of leakage may be by weight or by visual inspection. This test is of somewhat doubtful relevance to microbiological penetration.

Vials are a little less prone to pinhole cracks than ampoules. They are usually more robust and are not deliberately weakened in particular areas to allow opening. The main concern with vials is the integrity of the seal between the vial itself and its elastomeric closure.

Some degree of evaluation of the microbiological integrity of the vial/closure system can be made from the specified characteristics of the two components. In the first instance it would be reasonable to have a clear picture of the quality characteristics of the vial flange and the vial neck that affect container/closure integrity; concurrently to have a clear picture of the quality characteristics of the closure.

Closures may be flat discs or wads that rest on the vial, making contact with the flange, and being held in place by an overseal. This type of presentation is not used commonly nowadays, having been replaced in the main by plugs that fit into the neck of the vial (Fig. 2). These plugs also make contact with the flange of the vial and are held in place by an overseal.

The factors that ensure microbiological integrity are

(a) An interference fit between the outside diameter of the plug and the inside diameter of the vial neck. Any ovality within the vial neck may have an adverse effect on interference, but this may be compensated by distortion of the plug which is in turn a function of the composition of the elastomer. The finish of the two mating surfaces may also bear some influence.

(b) The completeness of the seal between the top surface of the flange of the vial and the bottom surface of the flange of the closure. This is affected by the compression forces exerted by the overseal and the elasticity of the closure. The finish of the two mating surfaces is of major importance.

It is generally understood that the principal means of ensuring the microbiological integrity of vial container/closure systems is via the two mating flanges. Morton et al. [7] studied container/closure characteristics by measuring the rate of pressure decay from sealed vials. Although relating directly to molecular

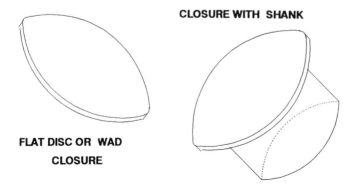

CLOSURE WITH SHANK

FLAT DISC OR WAD
CLOSURE

Fig. 2 Types of vial closure.

leakage from vials, the conclusions drawn by these workers are by inference applicable also to microbiological integrity. The most important factor contributing to container/closure integrity was the compression force applied by the overseal. Various differences in elastomeric properties of closures and defects in the surface finish of flanges could be compensated by closure compression.

Evaluation of the compression forces applied by overseals to sealed vials is therefore critical to the evaluation of microbiological integrity of glass vials with elastomeric closures. This ought to be determined at validation and monitored routinely in production. Equipment has been developed [8] to allow in-process measurement of the forces required to crimp overseals onto vial closures, thus revealing and automatically rejecting broken glass flanges, defective glass finishes, damaged or incorrect closures, etc.

It is not necessarily correct to assume that the neck fit is of no importance to microbiological integrity of vials. It may rather be of secondary importance to mating flanges. Interference is clearly of importance, for instance, to the microbiological integrity of prefilled syringes, where there are no mating flange surfaces. The primary microbiological seal in the prefilled syringe is effected by interference between the outside diameters of two or three ribs molded into the elastomeric plungertip and the inside diameter of the syringe barrel.

Other physical tests may allow routine in-place evaluation of the microbiological integrity of vials. Headspace gas analysis is one such method. Many sterile products are held under nitrogen or some other gas in vials. The gas content of the headspace should, with a perfect seal, remain constant over time rather than becoming equilibrated with the atmosphere under a less than perfect seal. This type of analysis is amenable to chemical methodology and is likely done routinely in pharmaceutical production for reasons other than evaluation of microbiological integrity.

The evaluation of vial seal integrity may also be done routinely by similar differential pressure measurement methodology to that used experimentally by Morton et al. [7]. The principle of the method is to detect leakage through the container/closure interface by reducing the pressure in an inspection head that surrounds the suspect region. Any change in pressure (leakage outward) from the item under test is detected by comparison with a blank for which no pressure change is possible. A fully automated 100% inspection system allowing automatic rejection has been described [9].

C. Flexible Containers

The solid contents of a flexible package containing a sterilized medical device are very unlikely to be small enough to leak out through a pinhole in the system of containment and be immediately noticeable. Yet pinholes are all that is needed to compromise the sterility of the product. The two issues surrounding flexible containers are the quality of the material and the quality of the seals.

The choice of materials of containment for flexible containers is of first importance. Waterproof materials are to be preferred in recognition of the potential for microorganisms to grow through damp materials that might otherwise have been resistant to penetration. Most materials are manufactured as continuous films or webs that, taking paper as an example, may be a few meters wide and very many meters in length. Variation in quality may occur across the width and along the length of the web. Random sampling to verify the quality is impossible once webs are wound up as cylindrical rolls. Some areas of web may be thinner or thicker than others, some stronger or weaker; some parts of the web may contain pinholes.

It is important to avoid the use of materials that are intrinsically prone to the occurrence of pinholes. Thinner materials are more prone to pinholes than thicker materials. Single-ply films are of greater risk than laminated or coated films because coatings fill in pinholes and because the probability of pinholes coinciding between two laminants is remote. Lamination may also add to the strength of a material so that pinholes do not occur during movement or as a consequence of pressure differentials in sterilization or transportation.

Detection of pinholes in flexible packaging is therefore an important aspect of the physical evaluation of their potential to maintain microbiological integrity. It is usually a specialized activity left to the manufacturers of packaging films.

According to various types of flexible containment systems for sterile medical products, there is a need to address the microbiological integrity of the seals. Some seals may be intended to be permanent, others openable. For instance a device may be packaged and sealed prior to sterilization into a two-piece pouch of say spun-bonded polyolefin and a transparent laminate, in which three sides of the pouch are permanently sealed and the fourth is intended to be opened (Fig. 3). The permanent seals may be double or triple or folded over to ensure integrity; the risky seal is the one that is intended to be opened. Another type of package might again be of two pieces, one transparent web preformed into a "blister" into which the device is placed, and a second flat web of paper bearing the printed instructions for use, being sealed to the blister on all four sides (Fig. 4). This type of packaging is used currently and widely for large-volume sterile medical devices such as hypodermic syringes and needles. All four seals are equally at risk, because any three have to be peeled apart to remove the device.

The primary method of physically evaluating seals is by their strength. The stronger the seal, the less likely it is to tear apart in sterilization, transport, or storage. Seal strength is defined as the force required to break apart a seal when the force is applied at right angles to the direction of the seal. Seal strength should be evaluated during validation and monitored during routine production. Sealing equipment has complexities that cannot be allowed to compromise the maintenance of sterility. Seals that are required to be opened should also be

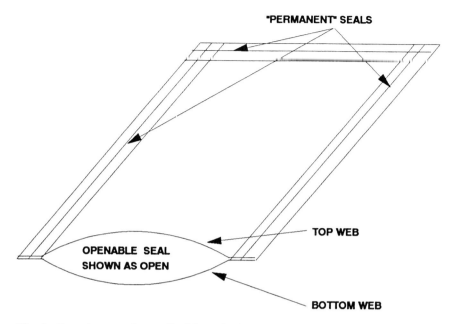

Fig. 3   Two-piece pouch-type flexible packaging.

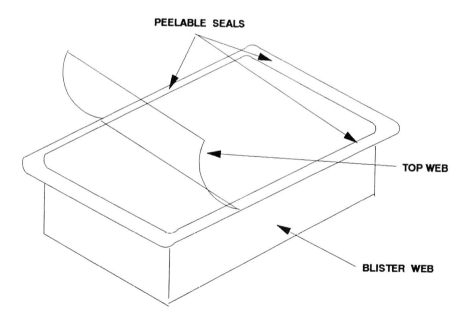

Fig. 4   Two-piece blister-type flexible packaging.

evaluated for so-called "peel strength." This is the force required to break apart a seal when applied in the same direction as the seal. This should obviously not be too high.

Another quantitative method of evaluating seal integrity is done with either filled and sealed packages or empty sealed packages. The air pressure differential method involves filling the package with air through a hollow needle until something "gives." Usually the package bursts along a seal. With commercially available equipment, seals can be evaluated at controlled rates of airflow into the package, and quantitative measures can be obtained of the pressure at which the seal bursts. This type of equipment also allows the determination of the weakest point around the seals and may thus help identify problems within the sealing equipment. It would be unusual for the web to be weaker than the seals, but this type of equipment can identify problems of this nature with appropriate modification.

Beyond these tests there are other cruder methods of evaluating seals for physical integrity. In a modification of the U.S. Federal Standard method for vials, there may be some information to be gained by placing a known volume of a liquid (say a 1% solution of methylene blue) into a flexible container in contact with its seals and allowing it to hang unsupported for a period of time. Leakage may be determined by dye penetration. Water resistant packs may be tested by slowly squeezing a pack immersed under water; leakage will be revealed by appearance of air bubbles. "Worst case" simulation methods may be applied to intact packs using particles of carbon black; this type of testing usually involves repeated cycles of pressure change simulating the sterilization process and worse; penetration is indicated by evidence of carbon black on the inside of the pack.

With all their limitations, these physical methods are better suited to flexible packaging than microbiological methods. They are, however, destructive.

REFERENCES

1. Parenteral Drug Association (1983). Technical Information Bulletin No. 4. *Aspects of Container/Closure* Integrity.
2. Frieben, W. R., Folck, R. J., and Devisser, A. (1982). Integrity testing of vial closure systems used for parenteral products. *Journal of Parenteral Science and Technology* **36**: 112–115.
3. Odlaug, T. E. (1984). Microbiological validation of container closure systems. *Pharmaceutical Manufacturing* **1**: 30–35.
4. Powell, D. B. (1972). Packaging of sterile medical products. In *Industrial Sterilization* (G. Briggs Phillips and W. S. Miller, eds.). Durham, N.C.: Duke University Press.
5. Reich, R. R. (1986). Packaging films: A method of microbial barrier evaluation. *Medical Device and Diagnostic Industry* **8**: 19–21.

6. Tallentire, A., and Sinclair, C. S. (1985). Microbiological barrier properties of uncoated and coated spunbonded polyolefin (Tyvek). *Medical Device and Diagnostic Industry* **7**; 50–54.

7. Morton, D. K., Lordi, N. G., and Ambrosio, T. J. (1989). Quantitative and mechanistic measurements of parenteral vial container/closure integrity by leakage quantitation. *Journal of Parenteral Science and Technology* **43**: 88–97.

8. Connor, J. T. (1983). In-process verification of closure seal integrity. *Journal of Parenteral Science and Technology* **37**: 14–19.

9. Khan, S. (1989). Automatic flexible aseptic filling and freeze-drying of parenteral drugs. *Pharmaceutical Technology* **13**: 24–34.

10
Parametric Release and Other Regulatory Issues

Sterility knows no frontiers. Sterile products are manufactured in all countries; they are used within national boundaries, they are imported, and they are exported. However, most governments will not permit the marketing of sterile pharmaceutical products or medical devices unless the products have been notified to them, scrutinized for safety and efficacy, and approved. It is not the intention of this chapter to describe in detail the activities of governmental authorities throughout the world in relation to sterile products but to draw attention to some of the issues that are peculiar to sterile products and sterilization.

The greatest amounts of governmental activity in the regulation of medical products are in the U.S.A. and in Europe. More often than not, the regulation of sterile products in other continents and countries tends to follow U.S. or western European models.

I. THE PHARMACOPOEIAS

Historically, the control of pharmaceutically active products has rested with the pharmacopoeias. Pharmacopoeias in one guise or other have been published since antiquity [1]. With the beginnings of greater mobility of commerce in the seventeenth and eighteenth centuries, local treatises on the purity of medicinal substances began to take on national stature, for instance the London Pharmacopoeia of 1618, the Pharmacopoeia Danica of 1772, etc. The first edition of the United States Pharmacopeia (USP) of 1820 predates the first British Pharmacopoeia (BP) of 1864.

Interest in international pharmacopoeial standards was taken up by the World Health Organization's International Pharmacopoeia of 1952 and its subsequent revisions. This differs from national pharmacopoeias in that it has no legal authority. Within the beginnings of the development of what is now the European Community, a European Pharmacopoeial Convention was signed in 1964, by whose terms the signatories undertook to make the standards of the European Pharmacopoeia (EP) the official standards of their countries. The majority of countries in western Europe are now signatories.

National pharmacopoeias, and EP, have legal status. They are legally constituted compendia of standards, some of which are mandatory and some of which are not. Taking the USP as an example, the pharmacopoeia is divided into monographs and General Chapters. The first purpose of the pharmacopoeias is to publish monographs. These are official specifications for drugs or devices. It is illegal for an item that is alleged to meet the requirements of a USP monograph to fail to do so. A product specified as being sterile in a pharmacopoeial monograph is required to be capable of passing the *Test for Sterility*. The *Test for Sterility* is not described in a monograph; it is described in a General Chapter. The BP and the EP are structured in the same way.

The General Chapters of the USP may be mandatory or nonmandatory. The mandatory chapters are themselves standards that define official "referee" test methods intended to be used in the event of litigation or arbitration concerning the status of items alleged to comply with the requirements of particular monographs. The *Test for Sterility* is a mandatory test. This does not in law mean that there is any obligation on a manufacturer to use the *Test for Sterility* as a release test or as part of a quality control/assurance program, although many do.

Table 1 Achieving Sterility in the Major Compendia

British Pharmacopoeia (1982)	
General Notices	For aqueous preparations, heating in an autoclave is the method of choice. The use of an alternative procedure is not precluded
Appendices	Test for Sterility (Appendix XVI)
	Methods for Sterilization (Appendix XVIII)
European Pharmacopoeia	
Annexes	Test for Sterility (Annexe VIII.3)
Methods of Preparation	Methods of Sterilization (Methods of Preparation IX.I)
United States Pharmacopeia (1990)	
General Chapters	<1> Injections—preparations for injections meet the requirements under Sterility Tests <71>
	<71> Sterility Tests
	<1211> Sterilization and Sterility Assurance of Compendial Articles

The nonmandatory General Chapters are not standards in the strictest sense, only guidelines, information, etc. They are frequently interpreted as being "best practice," and it can often make more economic sense to comply with their guidance than to take an alternative approach requiring the demonstration of equivalence or better. Within the USP there is a nonmandatory informational chapter entitled "Sterilization and Sterility Assurance of Compendial Articles," which outlines the concepts and principles involved in controlling the quality of allegedly sterile items.

Table 1 compares the structures of the USP, the EP, and the BP in their separate ways of dealing with sterile products. All three major compendia bear a close resemblance to one another.

II. GOOD MANUFACTURING PRACTICES

In modern times the control of both sterile and nonsterile medical products has moved beyond the scope of the pharmacopoeias alone and into the arena of governmental regulatory bodies. This is not to say that the pharmacopoeias do not still play a major part in the control of medical products. Regulatory agencies have found that they function best by having standards officially recognized for products rather than having to deal with separate specifications and analytical methodologies for each new registration. Nonetheless, governmental agencies may, in the best interests of the health of the community, wish to make new products available before public standards are published in the pharmacopoeias (the USP, for instance, is published in revision every five years). In these instances, official permission to market a product may predate its recognition by the pharmacopoeias.

Furthermore, in addition to the compendial restrictions on end-product specifications and referee tests, a need has been found for legal weapons extending into the ways and means by which products are manufactured. Regulatory agencies are justifiably concerned that particular drug substances may, if manufactured by a different method from that used for the original product on which the pharmacopoeial monograph was based, contain undesirable impurities that are not defined in the monograph. The U.S. Food, Drug and Cosmetic Act of 1938 gave the FDA the authority to inspect manufacturing facilities. The 1962 Kefauver-Harris amendments to the Act provided authority for publication of Good Manufacturing Practice Regulations in the U.S.A.

This movement to governmental regulation has led to publication of a range of governmental rules and guidelines affecting the manufacture of medical products. The main sources of regulations are, in the U.S.A., the *Code of Federal Regulations*, which publishes, in title 21, the basic requirements for registration of new drugs (the NDA or New Drug Application) and the Good Manufacturing Practice (GMP) Regulations for medical devices (Section 820) and pharmaceuticals (Section 821); in Europe, EEC *Guide to Good Manufacturing Practice for Pharmaceuticals* [2] and the U.K. "Blue Guide" [3] for sterile medical devices.

The U.S. *Code of Federal Regulations* has the force of law. As such, the U.S. GMPs are rather stark in their style and content. Two U.K. documents that have been of significant influence on the development of standards in Europe, the "Blue Guide" [3] and the "Orange Guide" [4], differ from the *Code of Federal Regulations* in that they have no statutory force. As such, their content (within three revisions of the Orange Guide, in 1971, 1977, and 1983, and two revisions of the Blue Guide, in 1981 and 1990) has always been more user-friendly. The EEC *Guide to Good Manufacturing Practice* [2] has arisen from an EEC Directive. The purpose of an EEC Directive is to set out principles and criteria that must be embodied in the national laws of the member states, and so the EEC guide [2] will have, in due course, the force of law for pharmaceutical GMPs throughout Europe. The EEC guide, however, has retained the user-friendly style of its origins in the Orange Guide. It has yet to be seen how legal authority will affect this in the future.

The Blue Guide is the only one of the pivotal regulatory documents that is particular to sterile products ("Sterile Medical Devices and Surgical Products"). In its 1990 revision, it has adopted the principles, style, and content of International (ISO 9000 to 9004), European (EN 29000 to 29004), and British Standards Organizations (BS 5750) requirements for integrated quality assurance systems. Additional requirements specific to sterile products are included.

The movement of the Blue Guide toward the ISO 9000 series of standards is an unusual example of convergence between quality assurance of medical and pharmaceutical products and quality assurance in other industries. The ISO 9000 series of standards is becoming the accepted norm for progressive customer-oriented companies in both western and eastern Europe. It rests on three important themes, which if addressed properly will provide a systematic basis to quality assurance:

(a) sufficient attention being given to product specifications, so that all products are suited to, and fit for, their intended purpose;

(b) an approach to quality that is comprehensive to all aspects of a product and its manufacture;

(c) formal documentation comprehensively defining and describing the organizations and procedures existing in a company to create and assure quality.

These themes of the ISO standards in no way contradict the themes that have been emphasized in the earlier and parallel pharmaceutical and medical devices GMP Regulations and Guides. Indeed many pharmaceutical companies are already putting pressure on their suppliers to gain accreditation with the ISO 9000 series of standards. It is possible that the way forward for GMPs in the sterile products manufacturing industry as a whole may eventually defer to these standards in the way of the Blue Guide.

Like the original U.K. guide to pharmaceutical GMP (the Orange Guide), the Blue Guide has no statutory force.

None of these official standards have ever been specific enough to be free from interpretative differences. As a consequence, to avoid embarrassment, to harmonize, and to educate, a number of voluntary and semiofficial bodies have over the years published "Best Practice," "Recommendations," "Guidelines," and even standards for the manufacture of sterile products. Many of these have been referred to in earlier chapters.

The Parenteral Drug Association (PDA) has led in offering guidance to the manufacture of sterile pharmaceuticals in the U.S.A., and its publications have been widely influential throughout the world. The FDA has itself been of considerable assistance in the publication of its own interpretative guidelines. To some extent this has been to provide the inspection branch with a basis for consistency in areas of scientific and technological disagreement. These guidelines have a similar status to the nonmandatory chapters of the pharmacopoeias; it is often easier to comply with the FDA by adopting their recommendations than to justify and argue equivalence. The need for these guidelines argues against the primary value of statutory regulation of technological matters.

In the area of sterile medical devices, the principal U.S. voluntary standards bodies have been the Health Industry Manufacturers' Association (HIMA) and the Association for the Advancement of Medical Instrumentation (AAMI). Other bodies working in the area of standards for sterile products and sterilization technologies include the American National Standards Institute (ANSI) and the International Standards Organization (ISO). The interactions of the various bodies involved in preparing standards is complicated, fluid, and not uncomplicated by political undertones. Some harmonization of these diverse activities occurred in 1989 with the AAMI, under the auspices of the ISO, being endorsed by the FDA, the HIMA, and the ANSI as the organization that should lead standards development in several medically related areas including sterilization technologies. It is likely that sterilization standards already published or to be published by the ISO Technical Committee 198 will be considered state-of-the-art by the FDA [5].

In Europe, sterile medical device legislation is to be published in 1993 to 1994 to allow the free passage of goods across national borders. The key to this legislation is "harmonized" standards. A list of harmonized standards is to be published in the "Official Journal of the European Communities," and manufacturers who comply with these harmonized standards will be presumed to comply with the statutory requirements. Harmonized standards for sterile products will have to be endorsed by the European Standards Organization (CEN) under the auspices of Technical Committee 204. CEN technical subcommittees are actively working in the area of medical device sterilization standards; in other areas such as GMP they have agreed to adopt the voluntary standards of the European Confederation of Medical Suppliers Associations (EUCOMED). This will certainly improve the confusing mish-mash of standards that have in the past existed in Europe.

The safety of the patient is the issue at stake when debating free trade and movement of sterile products across national and international borders. A good understanding of the alternative ways of meeting the same end is the basis of harmonization, and significant progress is being made in Europe and the U.S.A. separately and to a lesser extent between the two continents. National governments have a responsibility to protect the health of their populace, and differences in legislation will always arise according to the balance of expectations that exist between governments and industry in differing cultures.

III. THE FDA'S PREFERENCE FOR TERMINAL STERILIZATION

In the Federal Register of October 11, 1991, the FDA formally proposed that a rule should be established whereby aseptic processing of allegedly sterile pharmaceuticals should only be justifiable on the basis of the product being proven to be unsuitable for terminal sterilization. On ratification of the rule and after a phasing-in period of 18 months, manufacturers wishing to pursue aseptic processing of a new or existing sterile product must provide documentary evidence to the FDA of the product's unsuitability for terminal sterilization. Manufacturers requiring to change their existing aseptic processes to terminal sterilization will have their regulatory documentation fast-tracked through the FDA's bureaucracy. The rule was expected to be published in the Federal Register sometime in 1992.

The reaction of the pharmaceutical industry was so lukewarm to the proposal that 1992 and 1993 passed without ratification. This is not to say that the FDA has reconciled itself to shelving the rule; indeed, the inspection branch is placing greater and greater pressure on aseptic manufacturers toward stricter and stricter compliance with FDA guidelines and policy statements that in law have no authority. It would not be uncommon to see seemingly minor technical concerns like the failure of a laboratory to use magnification and illumination aids for plate counts cited alongside the absence of adequate validation protocols in the same FDA inspection reports (form 483). There is little doubt that the FDA is so convinced of the correctness of its view that it will continue to pursue the elimination of aseptic manufacture unless there is a step change improvement in available technology.

In making this proposal, the FDA recognizes that a dual standard of sterility assurance has been in operation. Terminal sterilization processes for parenteral pharmaceutical products are currently required to be validated to sterility assurance levels of 10^{-6}; aseptic processes can only be demonstrated to achieve sterility assurance levels of 10^{-3}. This is clearly an example of dual standards. Furthermore, to the FDA it appears to be fundamentally wrong for products that are quite capable of tolerating terminal sterilization to be manufactured aseptically.

In practical terms, terminal sterilization of liquid parenteral products means sterilization by saturated steam. Production of free radicals in water prohibits the application of radiation sterilization to aqueous products, but radiation sterilization may be suitable for some solid dosage forms. Dry heat and ethylene oxide are unlikely to be of any value. In the first instance, therefore, saturated steam should be the process of first choice for sterilization of thermally stable drug substances; dosage forms should not be formulated in ways that compromise thermal stability.

Beyond the ways in which the proposal affects drug substances and dosage forms, there are some uncertainties associated with various presentations. For instance, the FDA exempts prefilled syringes from their proposal, alleging that they are unsuitable for terminal sterilization. This is not necessarily true with all technologies, for instance sterilization by steam in ballasted autoclaves.

Moreover, some pharmaceutical products may be contained in plastics or other terminal sterilization labile materials. It is not clear whether the choice of materials for containers is sufficient justification to retain aseptic processing for dosage forms capable of withstanding terminal sterilization. The assessment of acceptability in such circumstances has been stated [6] to be based on demonstrable evidence that the particular package or container is of positive benefit to the patient. Some tricky decisions are likely to arise in this area.

The impact of the proposal may reopen a debate on the way in which SALs appear to be applied to aseptic processing. The origins of the SAL concept lie in terminal sterilization and rest heavily on the extrapolated effects of uniform sterilization treatments to populations of contaminants defined in terms of resistance and of numbers of contaminants (bioburden). The process of aseptic manufacture is a process of contamination control; the frequency of occurrence of a contaminated item within a population of aseptically filled items is a measure of bioburden, not a measure of the SAL. The SAL is the probability of those contaminants surviving, and this is a function of the types of contaminants and the formulation of the product. Formulations can be made to be antimicrobial. In principle this is no different from chemical sterilization.

If this principle is extended, then SALs of 10^{-6} may be attainable by aseptic manufacture followed by mild heat treatment.

All manufacturers seeking approval of new sterile products will need a strategy to justify the method of sterilization, terminal or aseptic or something in between. The technology chosen should minimally jeopardize the chemical, physical, and pharmacological properties of the dosage forms. Most cases are not going to be "open and shut," and the FDA and the industry have an interesting time ahead developing these strategies and decision-making processes.

IV. PARAMETRIC RELEASE

There are various definitions of parametric release, for instance

(a) . . . a sterility release procedure based upon effective control, monitoring, and documentation of a validated sterilization process cycle in lieu of release based upon end product sterility testing (FDA Compliance Policy Guide, 1987, Chapter 32a Parametric Release—Terminally Heat Sterilized Drug Products).

(b) . . . use of a specified set of engineering and microbiological data . . . to determine that a desired sterility assurance level is provided and maintained without the need of finished product sterility testing (Parenteral Drug Association Technical Report No. 8, 1987, Parametric Release of Parenteral Solutions Sterilized by Moist Heat Sterilization).

Whatever definitions may have been proposed by regulatory bodies and other committees for whatever specific purposes or processes, parametric release concerns eliminating end-product compendial sterility testing as the final criterion required to release sterile products. All of the major compendia recognize the severe statistical and technical limitations of the test for sterility. The test is formally acknowledged in the USP and the EP as a "referee test" in cases where there may be a dispute over sterility (or more likely nonsterility). So where are the barriers to parametric release?

A. Barriers to Parametric Release

The barriers to parametric release are complex, partly legal, partly historical or traditional, and muddled by issues of consistency.

The consistency issues are those of consistency among the various methods of achieving sterility (should some be eligible for parametric release while others should not be eligible?) and consistency among the sterility test and the various end-product chemical and physical tests required to release pharmaceutical products to market.

Among the four principal methods of achieving sterility (radiation, saturated steam, ethylene oxide, and aseptic filling), only one has been wholeheartedly accepted for parametric release: sterilization by gamma irradiation. End-product sterility testing has not been done on irradiated products for two decades. The justification for this lies in reliable knowledge of how microorganisms are killed by radiation, and in the reliability of the methods of process control and measurement of absorbed dose.

Sterilization by saturated steam has a longer history of practical application than irradiation, and the factors affecting microbial inactivation (temperature and time) are equally well known and thoroughly researched, yet parametric release for terminal sterilization by saturated steam has been addressed on paper far more regularly than it has been applied in practice. One barrier to parametric release for steam sterilization processes has been its technology. Steam sterilization has been around for a long time, and its technology is improving all the time; modern microprocessor-controlled autoclaves are pieces of very fine precision equipment, but there are many older, less well-controlled, autoclaves still in regular use. Patients have suffered and died from administration of nonsterile autoclaved products. Any mechanism therefore for allowing parametric release of steam sterilized products should emphasize the need for sound and reliable technology, but in doing this there is the danger of appearing to endorse the end-product sterility test as a justification for using unreliable technology that ought not to be used for sterilizing medical products in the first place. This is a paradox that can only be resolved through wider usage of parametric release for steam sterilized products, and indeed regulatory agencies might find parametric release a useful lever to force replacement or upgrading of obsolescent autoclaves.

Whereas radiation sterilization and steam sterilization technologies are clearly suitable for parametric release, ethylene oxide sterilization and aseptic filling are not thought to be suitable. Scientific knowledge of the interactions involved in ethylene oxide sterilization is less clear-cut than with radiation or steam. There is no agreement that aseptic filling can be shown to achieve comparable levels of sterility assurance to terminal sterilization processes. Therefore these two processes are not eligible for parametric release. The irony of this approach to parametric release is the intrinsic inconsistency of appearing to justify the release of products processed aseptically or by ethylene oxide sterilization on the basis of a test which we have "condemned" for better processes on the basis of it having statistical and technical limitations.

This lack of evident consistency has arisen from a long-standing debate over the value of product control versus process control. This is the main historical or traditional barrier to the introduction of parametric release.

Product control in its crudest sense is the notion of manufacturing a product any old way and then testing it to see whether it meets certain end-product specifications. The decision to release is based on the end-product test results. To some extent this is exactly how the sterility test is seen to be used in the decision-making process for the release of product, certainly as it applies to rejection of product. If a sample of a sterilized product fails to pass a sterility test then it is usually rejected regardless of how much confidence the manufacturer may have in data generated through sterilization validation studies, biological validation studies, sterilizer control, and routine monitoring programs. The FDA insists that if a *Sterility Test* failure cannot be positively attributed to laboratory contamination, it must be assumed to have arisen from a problem in the manufacturing process. This is a conservative one-tailed error, quite different from the thoughts that led to the inclusion of retests in the compendia, thoughts which concluded that sterility tests are so difficult to carry out that laboratories deserved an automatic right to retest.

Process control implies measurement of critical parameters of raw materials and intermediates as they are converted to finished products, and monitoring and controlling the critical process parameters that may influence finished product quality. Process control is what parametric release is all about. In processes where the level of reliability in process control can be predicted to be high, there is a sound basis for eliminating the sterility test. Where process control is not so reliable, the sterility test should be considered as one part of the armory of process control tests rather than as an overriding end-product test, in other words a Pass in the sterility test should never in these processes be allowed to overrule evident failure to meet all of the prescribed in-process test criteria.

The legal barrier to the introduction of parametric release is usually couched in terms of a question. In the event of a legal dispute over nonsterility how could you convince a jury that a batch of your product could pass a sterility test if you had never actually tested it?

B. The Price to Pay for Parametric Release

There is no such thing as a free lunch (Henry Ford). Eliminating the sterility test is not merely a technical issue; it has wide-ranging commercial implications. Release of many billions of dollars worth of pharmaceutical and medical products is held up each day while sterility tests are incubating. It should not be believed that parametric release leads to the realization of all of these costs.

The price of parametric release is in process control. The requirement to control processes is critical. There is no defence to the legal barrier discussed above if the sterility test is dropped in favor of process controls that are inadequate. Processes should not only be controlled but monitored, and there must be predetermined standards for process characteristics, and these standards must be met, or product must be rejected. Parametric release is an all-or-nothing condition—there is no way that a batch of product can be tested and released by an end-product sterility test if satisfactory process criteria are not met.

Among various monographs, guides, and recommendations to parametric release, all are agreed that the terminal sterilization process must be validated, controlled, calibrated, and monitored. There should be independent means of monitoring and recording critical parameters; data should be reviewed and decisions made by an independent quality control function. The bioburden on the product should also be controlled. In other words, all of the determinants of sterility must be addressed in a satisfactory manner.

By and large it is in the control of bioburden that opinions differ. Batch-by-batch sampling and monitoring of product bioburden prior to sterilization is one route. Much of the commercial advantage of parametric release is lost if this expedient is adopted. Without due attention to process control criteria, product bioburden control prior to sterilization is as statistically and technically flawed as end-product sterility testing.

Many recommendations refer to general codes of GMP for bioburden control. Most of these are less than specific. A practical approach is to address parametric release as an integral process from raw materials through terminal sterilization and on to the systems employed to maintain sterility.

As a beginning, manufacturers should analyze their processes and identify each system or control that may have an effect on bioburden. Figure 1 is a simplified and generalized example of an analysis of a process in which a product is aseptically filled and then terminally sterilized. Each system or control affecting microbiological contamination is identified within this schematic and categorized as critical, major, or minor. The nature of the classification is that failure of any one critical system or control versus its predetermined standard during manufacture must lead to rejection of the batch. Parametric release may be permitted with as many as one major parameter exceeding its limit or two minor parameters.

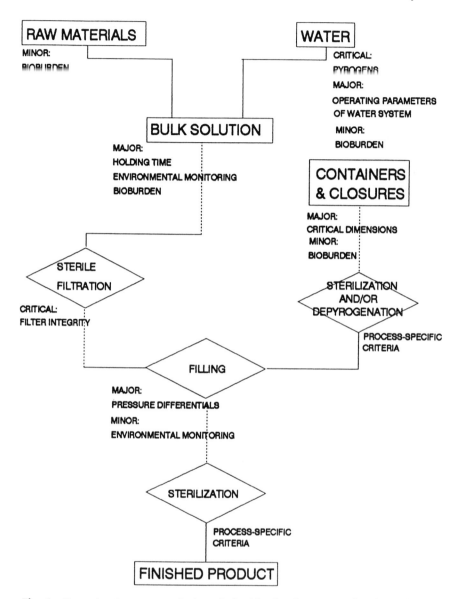

Fig. 1 Example of process analysis and classification for parametric release (aqueous filterable products).

The rationale of the classifications may best be seen by reference to products and processes with different levels of control. As a first example, the classification of holding times for bulk solutions and for microbiological monitoring shown in Fig. 1 as major apply to a product that is capable of supporting microbial growth; these could be relaxed to minor for inimical products.

As a second example, Fig. 2 is an analysis of a process in which the product cannot be passed through a sterilizing filter and for which the containers are not presterilized.

(a) In this process there is a critical classification given to the holding time for the bulk nonfilterable product prior to sterilization versus only a major classification for holding times for the sterile filtered product of Fig. 1. This is because the bioburden on the nonfilterable bulk may increase in numbers during an overlong holding period to an unacceptably high challenge for the terminal sterilization process.

(b) Bioburden on containers need only be classified as minor when they are presterilized, but it becomes of major importance when they are not. One process has a control measure (presterilization) in place and the other has not.

This type of approach recognizes that each manufacturer, each product, each facility, each process is unique. Therefore the criteria that have to be met must also be unique. It places a demand on a thorough and exhaustive analysis of process and on what, how, and where controls and monitoring points are applied. Even without a payoff from parametric release, it affords a disciplined approach to the manufacture of sterile products.

The lure of parametric release to commercial organizations is undoubtably monetary, either as reduced inventory costs or as reduced lead times within the supply chain. The cost balancing this out is better process control. From the standpoints of quality, sterility assurance, and responsibility to the recipient of the sterile product, the loss of a wholly inadequate end-product test is a low price to pay for more attention being given to the process characteristics that really influence sterility.

V. FDA PREAPPROVAL INSPECTION

The activities of the U.S. Food and Drug Administration have reverberations around the world. A major change to previously established custom and practice began in the early 1990s: the enforcement of inspection prior to granting approval to market a new product or a "significantly" changed product (preapproval inspection). Preapproval inspection is not a requirement unique to sterile products, but irrespective of that, it deserves to be specifically addressed

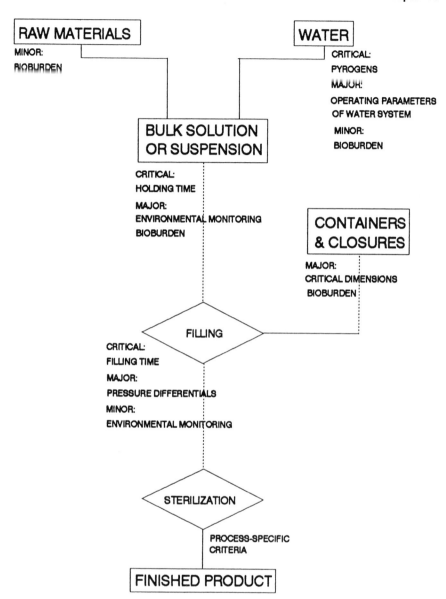

Fig. 2   Example of process analysis and classification for parametric release (nonfilterable products).

in this text. It is an activity that is taking place in relation to both pharmaceuticals and medical devices.

A. Preapproval Inspection for Pharmaceutical Products

The FDA's reputation for fairness and impartiality was dented in 1989 by scandal, corruption, and fraud. The pharmaceutical industry, particularly that part concerned with the manufacture of generic products, was also tainted. The FDA's backlash has been to move away from "systems of trust" toward strict enforcement of compliance. The linchpin of the FDA's new attitude has been preapproval inspection, incorporated into formal enforcement programs on October 1, 1990.

Before the introduction of preapproval inspection, the FDA undertook general inspections of manufacturers' facilities, procedures, and controls across the range of products that might be made in the same facility and against the GMP regulations (part 211 of the Code of Federal Regulations). Typically, approval would only be withheld if deficiencies found on inspection were significant enough to result in official regulatory action. The whole focus of inspection has now moved toward product-specific inspection, comparing in great depth the claims made in the New Drug Application (NDA) or amendment (ANDA) with the actual practices in the manufacturer's facilities, beginning with the facilities, procedures, and controls used in the manufacture of biobatches and ending with the facilities, procedures, and controls used in the manufacture of commercial batches. Parts 310, 312, 314, and 320 of the Code of Federal Regulations describe the basic requirements for NDAs. The inspection and review branches of the FDA are working together far more closely than ever before, and it is now usual for an inspector to bring his own copy of the relevant chapters of the NDA onto a manufacturer's premises at the time of inspection. Approval may be withheld even if formal regulatory action is not required.

Preapproval inspection has always been part of the FDA's armory of enforcement. Formerly it was commonly used only in connection with newly constructed facilities, or where existing facilities had never been inspected before, or where a period of two years had elapsed since a previous inspection on a similar dosage form. All of these criteria still apply, but all new chemical entities must be preapproved; for products currently being distributed, the top 200 are to be inspected for approval, and drugs with a narrow therapeutic range are to be preapproved.

B. Preapproval Inspection for Medical Devices

The level of scrutiny given by the FDA to medical devices is less than that given to pharmaceutical products. Inspection is, as always with the FDA, thorough. Most medical device manufacturers, however, are not subject to premarket inspection. Their responsibility to the FDA is in the main through a premarket notification process (510k) in which they must demonstrate substantial equivalency of their device to existing devices with respect to intended purpose, efficacy, safety, and essential technological characteristics. Devices with new applications are subject to a premarket approval (PMA) process.

The PMA process requires it to be demonstrated that a device has clinical utility. The idea of clinical utility goes beyond safety and efficacy; it means that a device is capable of providing clinically significant results. Kahan [7] illustrates this simply by reference to a hypothermia device. The intended purpose of the hypothermia device is to heat tissue. The device may be used in cancer treatment. Little is known of the therapeutic benefit of hypothermia devices to the treatment of cancer. Premarket approval for a hypothermia device based on a new technology approval would require data indicating clinically significant results from the use of the device in the treatment of cancer.

Recent legislation in the U.S.A., the Safe Medical Devices Act of 1990, has increased the range of types of devices required to go through the premarket approval process rather than the premarket notification (510k) process. This may be indicative of future FDA activity in the devices sector along the lines seen with pharmaceutical products.

REFERENCES

1. Grainger, H. S. (1981). The pharmacopoeias: Their origins and functions. In *Progress in the Quality Control of Medicines* (P. B. Deasy and R. F. Timoney, eds.) London: Elsevier Biomedical Press.
2. Commission of the European Communities (1992). *The Rules Governing Medicinal Products in the European Community, Volume IV. Guide to Good Manufacturing Practice for Medicinal Products.* Luxembourg: Office for Official Publications of the European Communities.
3. U.K. Department of Health (1990). *Quality Systems for Sterile Medical Devices and Surgical Products 1990. Good Manufacturing Practice.* London: Her Majesty's Stationery Office.
4. U.K. Department of Health and Social Security (1983). *Guide to Good Pharmaceutical Manufacturing Practice 1983.* London: Her Majesty's Stationery Office.
5. Chamberlain, V. C. (1992). U.S. GMP Requirements and ISO Development Status. In *Bioburden in Medical Device and Surgical Dressing Manufacture, Conference Proceedings.* Brussels: EUCOMED.
6. Frieben, W. (1990). Process development issues for sterile products: Strategy for selecting a sterile manufacturing technology. In *Proceedings of the PDA/PMA Sterilization Conference, August 26-29, 1990.* Washington, D.C.
7. Kahan, J. S. (1991). Clinical utility and medical device premarket approval. *Medical Device and Diagnostic Industry* **13**: 62–64.

Index